# Alzheimer Solutions

## A Personal Guide for Caregivers

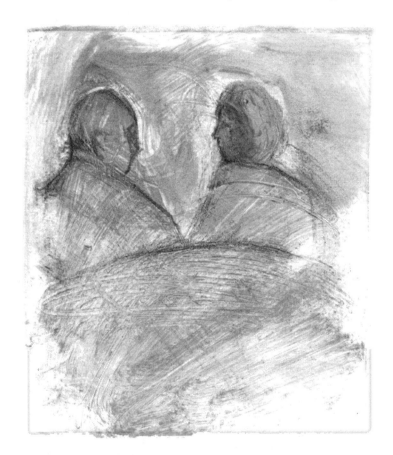

## By Jim Knittweis and Judith Harch

*Lucid Press*
*Sausalito, California*
*2002*

*Library of Congress Cataloging-in-Publication Data*

Knittweis, Jim, 1946-
    Alzheimer solutions: a personal guide for caregivers / Jim Knittweis & Judith Harch.
        p.   cm.
Includes biographical references and index
        ISBN 0-9646184-5-1 (alk. Paper)
        1. Alzheimer's disease—Patients—Care—Popular works. I. Harch, Judith, 1944- II.
Title
RC523.2.K65 2002
616.8'31—dc21                                        All Rights Reserved
                            2001050786

Cover design:  Vince Valdes
Editor: Robert I. Greenberg
Artist: Jenette Foster, Monotype
Copy Editor: A. Ranney Johnson

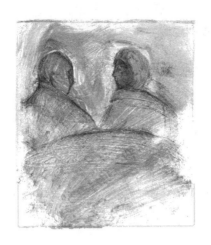

# Alzheimer Solutions
# A Personal Guide For Caregivers

## CONTENTS

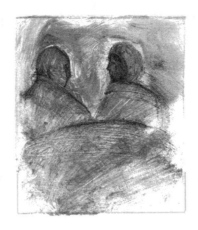

# INTRODUCTION

Alzheimer caregivers need help and they need it quickly. Quite often, this demanding role is a first-time experience for many who suddenly find themselves as the primary source of comfort and security for an ailing loved one. As a caregiver, you may have already discovered that dealing with basic day-to-day patient care while maintaining your own sense of self is a daily challenge.

The luxury of free time to read, research, or seek solutions to new problems is one that an Alzheimer caregiver can't afford. Caregivers need answers to a myriad of questions but don't always have time to find them. They need solutions that jump off the page of a book.

In ALZHEIMER SOLUTIONS – *A Personal Guide For Caregivers*, we've combined Jim Knittweis' problem-solving skills learned during his own caregiving experience with Judith Harch's non-technical, journalistic style. The question and answer format will help you easily locate information according to its relevance to your life. You can rely on the book as a quick reference for recurring or new problems as they arise.

The solutions we offer were collected over a 10-year period. They are derived from Jim Knittweis' firsthand experience during the years he looked for ways to not only care for his father's physical needs, but to bring small joys to a diminishing life.

Solutions also came from conversations with members of Alzheimer support groups and associations, caregivers and their families, and research findings from the medical community. Jim Knittweis created and has maintained the website ALZHEIMER

SOLUTIONS (**www.caregiving-solutions.com**) since 1999. His site is highly interactive. He encourages feedback from the many caregivers who visit. We've listened to those caregivers. We know which questions they want answered. We understand that the intensive day-to-day care required of an Alzheimer patient is the foundation of a caregiver's concern and the cause of caregiver burden.

Our book is not meant as a guide to the latest medical information about the disease. This is an exciting time full of promise in the field of Alzheimer's research! Any medical advances we might mention could quickly become obsolete. To help keep you current on the latest discoveries, we've included an appendix containing a listing of highly reputable resources, including many Internet websites.

Additionally, you will find a list of suggested readings from the Alzheimer's Association's Public Publications Catalog at the end of each chapter. The catalog is available by contacting the association at 800-272-3900. It lists many brochures, pamphlets, and fact sheets on a wide range of subjects. These materials are brief, fact filled, and a great resource for time-starved caregivers. They are available free or at low cost through local chapters. We've used the 2001 edition of the catalog.

When caregivers learn to deal effectively with difficult behavior problems, placement of their loved one into a nursing home can often be delayed. If that is your goal, the information in our book will be of great value toward meeting that goal.

If nursing home placement becomes necessary for your patient, you will be faced with a difficult task. Many caregivers don't know where or when to begin their search for the right nursing home. Appendix C – *Choosing a Nursing Home* offers many suggestions to help you start that important search.

Alzheimer's disease has come to the forefront of the American healthcare arena. A wealth of information and support is out there waiting for you. Take advantage of all that is offered. You are not in this alone. Help is yours for the asking. ALZHEIMER SOLUTIONS – *A Personal Guide For Caregivers* is a roadmap. Use it for this most challenging journey.

As you read our book, we hope you sense the compassion and respect we feel toward Alzheimer patients and their caregivers. Whether you volunteered for the job or had it thrust upon you, caregiving is a higher calling, a noble undertaking. May this book lighten your burden.

*Jim Knittweis and Judith Harch*

# FOREWORD

*By Joan Webb, RN, MSN*

After many years as a bedside nurse, I know that caring for a loved one with Alzheimer's disease is an enormous undertaking. In nursing as well as in home caregiving, each patient situation is unique and requires creativity, perseverance, and a team effort to find solutions that work. Sometimes, answers are clear and practical. Other times, simple answers seem elusive. I believe that the simple answers some-time elude us because it is difficult to grasp the true depth of memory loss in Alzheimer's dementia. Early in my career, I learned that lesson from the daughter of an Alzheimer patient.

Sarah, an elderly woman, had been admitted into the intensive care unit during the night with heart problems. She continually requested food from the moment she arrived. The night shift nurses had given her graham crackers and milk several times, but that didn't ease her hunger. When I served Sarah her breakfast tray, I thought the problem had been solved. But even though she ate the entire meal, the complaints of hunger did not go away. Throughout the morning, I, too, supplied her with graham crackers and milk to no avail. Her requests for food continued.

When Sarah's daughter arrived for a visit, she told me her mother's constant com-plaints of hunger had started several weeks previous to her hospital visit. It wasn't until her daughter began thinking at the most fundamental level that she realized the problem. Her mother was always hungry because she could no longer remember when she had last eaten. The daughter called on some creative thinking to come up with the solution. She began feeding her mother one food item at a time and inter-spersed the offering of food throughout the day along with the activities of daily living.

That afternoon, I followed the daughter's suggestion and stretched Sarah's lunchtime meal over several hours. Each request for food was met with a positive response, one piece at a time. By the time dinner trays arrived, I knew the daughter's solution was a success. My patient's demands for food were now a pleasant part of our interaction.

In ALZHEIMER SOLUTIONS – *A Personal Guide For Caregivers*, Jim Knittweis and Judith Harch have created a reader-friendly book filled with practical solutions to the problems facing millions of caregivers each day. The authors share many of the same nursing "tricks of the trade" that I learned over time. Patient and caregiver problems and solutions are presented in an easy-to-follow question and answer format. The questions are written just as a caregiver might ask them, and the authors address the hands-on, day-to-day care required of Alzheimer patients. Each question is met with a list of practical solutions that will guide you on your journey and spark your cre-ative problem-solving abilities.

Jim Knittweis' personal journey as a primary caregiver to his father brings authenticity to the book. He has walked in your shoes and spent countless hours researching practical solutions to difficult problems. Judith Harch writes in a clear style that allows the reader to find quick, easy-to-understand answers that often elude those closest to the problem.

The information is presented in a format that will allow you to quickly find practical help without searching the whole book. You will inevitably encounter difficult days. I recommend that you read the entire book, and then keep it handy as a reference guide.

The emotional and physical well being of the caregiver also is addressed. As a nurse educator, I know the importance of caring for the caregiver. I constantly remind my students that the person holding their patient's hand is also in need of attention. Jim and Judith clearly explain this important fact in a way that both honors and respects the primary caregivers who shoulder the tremendous burden and the secondary caregivers who support those caregivers.

This is a book you will reach for again and again. Use it often for its practical solutions and for creative inspiration, as your patient's needs change. You are not alone in your journey. ALZHEIMER SOLUTIONS – *A Personal Guide For Caregivers* will be a resourceful companion.

*Joan Webb is a Clinical Nurse Specialist in Critical Care, has a Post-Master's Certificate in Community Nursing, and is a nursing instructor at Widener University.*

# About the Authors

**Researcher Jim Knittweis** has been academically and personally involved with Alzheimer disease for the past 10 years. He was a primary caregiver for his father who died of the disease and is the founder of Alzheimer Solutions, an e-commerce company that offers a line of products for caregivers to help patients live as comfortably as possible. He maintains and updates his website (www.caregiving-solutions.com) with the latest in medical research and breaking news and has designed an evaluation test for those concerned about developing Alzheimer's. Jim is a member of the Delaware Valley Geriatric Society and holds a Master's Certificate in Clinical Gerontology and a Bachelor of Arts Degree in Psychology. His papers have been published in *Neurology, Medical Hypotheses* and *The Journal of the American Geriatrics Society.*

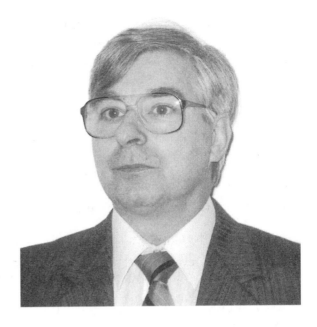

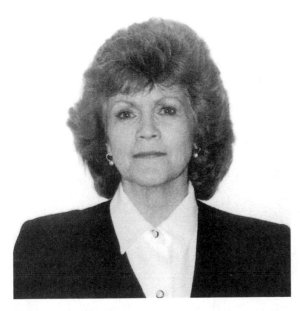

**Judith Harch** is a non-fiction freelance writer whose work appears in the *Philadelphia Inquirer.* She was a freelance columnist for the Camden (NJ) *Courier-Post* and a scriptwriter for *Comcast TV.* As a freelance nursing journal editor, she was Managing Editor of the publication *National Association of Orthopaedic Nurses Core Curriculum for Orthopaedic Nursing* (NAON)*, a Review Course* and Manuscript Reviewer for NAON's *Orientation to the Orthopaedic Operating Room* (1995). Her editing credentials include the medical journals *Clinical Research* (now titled *Journal of Investigative Medicine*) and the *Journal of Pediatric Ophthalmology & Strabismus* and as a contributing writer to the *Clinical Research* newsletter. Nursing journal editing credits include the nursing journals *Orthopaedic Nursing, Pediatric Nursing, ANNA Journal* and *Nursing Economics.*

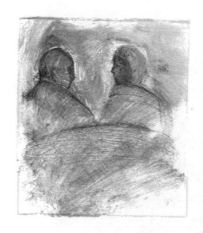

# ACKNOWLEDGMENTS

I dedicate this book to the memory of my father, Walter Knittweis, who taught me the meaning of compassion and to my mother Betty, who taught me the meaning of love and patience. Special thanks go to Whitney McMullen, gerontologist and close friend, for her help in collecting research materials for this book. I thank Jack Gomberg, MD, a masterful physician who directed my father's care during his years with Alzheimer's. And I would like to recognize the late Benjamin S. Frank, MD who encouraged my interest in biochemistry.

*Jim Knittweis*

First and best, I thank my husband, Chris, for his limitless patience and unwavering support. Two mentors helped pave the road that brought me to writing this book. Kaye Coraluzzo and Claudia Cuddy, wonderful friends, colleagues and accomplished medical journal managing editors, taught me all I know about the field. Their generosity, offered as the gift of time and the passing of knowledge, is the very definition of the word mentor.

*Judith Harch*

Both authors express their gratitude to Joan Webb for generously sharing her nursing wisdom and willingness to help us find the way to say it best. We thank Claire Huff for believing in us and Bob Greenberg for his editing expertise, always offered in the kindest manner. The Alzheimer's Association deserves special recognition. It could not have been more helpful. The organization's members stand ready to help all who ask. And an extra thanks goes to Brian Hance, Association Director of the Alzheimer's Associate *Safe Return* program.

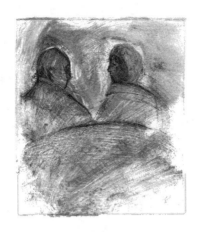

*~ "It is one of the most beautiful compensations of life, that
no man can sincerely try to help another without helping himself." ~*

Ralph Waldo Emerson

# PREFACE

The summer of 1990 was the last of many carefree summers at the shore with my dad. It was the year that Alzheimer's disease changed the lives of all those who loved my father, Walter Knittweis.

Since my childhood, our family vacation home on Long Beach Island, New Jersey has served as our gathering place. Our shore home sits along a beautiful bay. As a young-ster, summers meant lazy days of fishing and crabbing with my parents and brother, Walt, Jr. Even into my adulthood, our beach home brought memories of summers filled with home-cooked meals shared with extended family and cool, refreshing dips in the bay after hot, humid days spent fixing up the house. In 1990, my dad was a healthy, vigorous 77 years old. We had spent much of that summer repairing a broken bulkhead. Dad did the work of a person many years his junior, digging with shovels and hauling heavy boards. We worked side-by-side.

I've always enjoyed being with Dad. He was slight of build but had remarkable physical strength. When I was seven, I remember our working out together with barbells and weights. He loved to amaze me with his ability to lift me while I held onto my barbells. By the winter of 1990, it would become my turn to carry Dad. On a blustery November day, a foreboding fear that something was terribly wrong with Dad hit my mother Betty and me like the punch of a winter blizzard. As Mom and I watched TV that day, Dad suddenly stormed up from his basement workshop and demanded to know why I had stolen his hammer. I went downstairs with him to the workshop and showed him that the hammer was where it belonged. He seemed satisfied. A half-hour later, he returned to the living room obviously angry and agitated as he once again accused me of stealing his hammer. Nothing seemed to calm him. He stalked off to the workshop. Mom and I then heard great crashing and banging. Dad had taken a sledgehammer and had methodically broken every piece of machinery in his workshop. His treasured table saw lay in huge, torn chunks of twisted metal on the floor. I knew, intuitively, that something new, different and awful was happening. But I didn't know what it was.

Dad was immediately taken to Friends Hospital in Philadelphia for psychiatric evaluation. Our worst fears were realized when he was diagnosed with Alzheimer's disease. We were stung by those frightening words. Like most families, shock and disbelief flooded over us. We were fortunate to have a personable, optimistic, young geriatric psychiatrist to help us through what lay ahead. Dr. Jack Gomberg became Dad's physician and our partner in care.

After two weeks under Dr. Gomberg's watchful eye, Dad was well enough to return home. We welcomed him back with a mixture of hopefulness and a fear of the un-known. A million questions about the challenge we were about to face fueled that fear. We were grateful that Dad no longer seemed to have the insight to realize what this disease would do to him. The next few years brought many days of relative tranquillity. Dad was sociable, friendly, and cooperative. At times, he seemed almost normal. He returned to tinkering in his workshop. When he, once again, asked about the hammer, I was prepared. I had solved that sticky situation by purchasing several hammers and placing them around the workshop so he could easily find one.

His memory had begun to fail, but at times, he could recall fond moments of the past with great clarity. One winter while my aunt was visiting, she began singing the words to a song from the Big Band era. Dad sang right along with her, remembering the exact lyrics. Therapists have told me that Alzheimer patients respond well to "reminiscence therapy," which encourages patients to recall events, people and special memories of the past. During the reign of Big Band music, my parents had gone dancing every week. Those precious memories clung tenaciously to my father's mind.

Dr. Gomberg constantly monitored and changed Dad's medications and dosages to keep life at home manageable. But the inevitability of decline was apparent. The first half of 1993 passed uneventfully. But during that summer, as we returned to Long Beach Island, all was not well. Dad enjoyed the sunshine but repeatedly said that he wanted to sell the shore house. He could give no apparent reason for this decision. In the past, he had made family financial decisions. But by this time, out of necessity, Mom had taken complete control of money matters. She held firm that the shore home would remain a sanctuary for the family.

Dad's decline moved in fast-forward that summer. His solo strolls through the neigh-borhood had come to an end. He could no longer remember which house was his and often knocked on neighbors' doors looking for home. He now had to be accompanied on his walks. Then he began having trouble recognizing my mom. One day as she sat at her desk at the shore house, he said to her, "Get away from that desk, it belongs to

Betty, my wife." Mom had become very resourceful and clever finding ways around Dad's lack of recognition of her. Whenever he accused her of being a stranger, Mom would leave by the back door. A few minutes later, she would arrive at the front door and greet Dad saying, "Hi Walt. It's Betty. I'm back." Each time, Dad was fooled by this ploy and happy once again to see his wife.

By late autumn 1993, our lives took an ominous turn. One day, I received an alarming call at work from my brother. In an agitated state, Dad had grabbed Mom's wrist and squeezed it hard enough to cause a blood vessel to burst. She was frightened and bleeding badly. Fortunately, the bleeding was stopped with a compress. Against his will, Dad was admitted to Friends Hospital. The incident left my mom shaken and afraid of my father. She was reluctant to visit him at the hospital because she feared that he would ask to come home.  My heart ached for her. This was the man she still loved deeply.

After two weeks at the hospital, Dad no longer remembered the awful incident. He was ready to come home, but the decision about nursing home placement was now pressing. Dr. Gomberg explained that Dad had advanced to a severe stage of dementia. It would be impossible to guarantee that another violent episode would not occur. Mom made the decision to place Dad in a nursing care facility. Other family members agreed.

The day before Dad's hospital discharge to the nursing home was the saddest day of my life. I looked into his warm, gentle face and knew in my heart that he would never return home. That evening at the hospital, Dad was very talkative. He recalled the great times we spent in Florida catching fish and shrimp in the Indian River. I wanted nothing more on that cold November night than to take his hand and spirit him off to sunny Florida one last time. But I knew it couldn't happen. Instead, I had to find a way to tell him where he was going the next day.

To this day, I cannot remember how I told him. But somehow I had managed to get those difficult words out. We were fortunate in our choice of facilities. The nursing home was a cheerful place with a wonderful staff. Dad adjusted to it better than we had expected. Each time we visited him, he was friendly, talkative and had actually gained some of his lost weight. Although he was doing well both physically and emotionally, I somehow knew that Dad was near the end.

My connection to my father was so strong I seemed to know without doubt that he would not be in the nursing home long. On the day of admittance, the social worker, with polite frankness, asked my mother how she would pay for the years of nursing home care my father would require. I remain bewildered at my response. I said to her, "I don't think it's going to be a problem because Dad is only going to be in here a month." Where did that thought come from? I still don't know. One month later, Dad unexpectedly became ill enough to be transferred back to the hospital. He suffered from severe vomiting and dehydration. Mom and I stayed with him until the close of visiting hours. I watched Mom as she tenderly held his hands, said "goodnight," and said we would see him early the next morning. He flashed me a beautiful smile, squeezed my hand tightly and said, "See you, Jim."

That night, I awoke from a deep sleep at 3:00 a.m. I am normally a heavy sleeper. A proverbial freight train could roll over me without my waking. But this night was profoundly different. When I awoke, I knew with a chilling certainty that Dad was dying. Sadly, I was right. The hospital reported that he had developed complications at about 3:00 a.m. and had passed away shortly after. I believe very strongly that my father reached across time and space to say goodbye to me one last time. After his death, my mother suffered tremendous guilt for placing Dad in a nursing home. Guilt often holds a tight grip on Alzheimer caregivers. My brother and I tried to help Mom understand that she had done the right thing at the appropriate time. We could not comfort her. One night I prayed to God that He would allow Dad to send my mom a sign that he understood and still loved her.

The following morning, I sat quietly drinking coffee with my mom. She began telling me that she had experienced a strange dream during the night. She dreamed that Dad had come to her as a young, good-looking, fashionably dressed man with the jet-black hair of his youth. He had smiled at her and simply said, "I love you." The dream brought great solace to my mother and a sense of closure to her grief.

Many families adjust to an Alzheimer's diagnosis in a similar way. First, there is shock and disbelief. Then the adjustment process begins. Some families seek additional medical opinions, others seek alternative medicines. Some families seek information and learn all they can about the disease. That was my way of coping.

When Dad was diagnosed in 1990, I began an intensive search to learn all I could about Alzheimer's. I returned to college to earn a Master's certificate in Gerontology and a certificate in Laboratory Biotechnology. I had hoped to find some obscure, forgotten therapy or a cure for this devastating disease. My search also included ways to make life more comfortable for my father. I looked for products that could help preserve his dignity as an adult living in a childlike state. My search and research culminated in ALZHEIMER SOLUTIONS – *A Personal Guide For Caregivers.* Then I gathered my collected information and looked for the person who could help me bring it all together in a reader-friendly book. I didn't have to look far. My co-author, Judith Harch, is married to my cousin. I knew of her many years as a newspaper columnist and medical journal editor. After several years and many brainstorming sessions, we offer you our solutions to the difficult and noble acts caregivers perform each day.

Dad always told me that I would write a book some day and that he would be very happy and proud when that day arrived. This is that book. It is dedicated to my father, Walter Knittweis. To my fellow caregivers, I wish you peace on your journey during the long goodbye. In difficult times, remember The Serenity Prayer:

*"God grant me the serenity to accept the things I cannot change,*
*the courage to change the things I can,*
*and the wisdom to know the difference."*

Jim Knittweis

# Chapter One

## Helping Your Patient
## With
## Activities of Daily Living

*~ "You will find as you look back upon your life that the moments when you have truly lived are the moments when you have done things in the spirit of love" ~*

Henry Drummond

# Dealing With Mealtime Problems

Alzheimer patients often exhibit unusual eating behaviors. Some aspects of these behaviors are physical in nature, some are related to the continuing process of dementia, and some are related to the loss of sensory perception.

We take for granted the relationship between hunger and how eating satisfies that feeling. But your patient may no longer remember that simple relationship. Your patient may forget where eating takes place, or how to use eating utensils. He or she may actually forget the physical process of chewing and swallowing.

Even the question of what can and should be eaten can become a source of danger. Vigilance on your part will be important to protect your patient from ingesting anything harmful.

A great deal of patience, an awareness that your loved one is in the process of unlearning the most fundamental lessons they've accumulated over a lifetime, and choosing your battles wisely, will help make mealtime more pleasant for you and your patient.

The following is a discussion of mealtime problems and suggested solutions. Instructions for the Heimlich maneuver also are included. The Heimlich maneuver is used on choking victims. Everyone can benefit from knowing this simple, potentially lifesaving procedure (preferably, before you need to use it). You may want to copy and post the instructions in your eating area.

### What activities may be distracting at mealtime? How can I eliminate or avoid these distractions?

- The need to "go to the bathroom" frequently is a mealtime distraction. Toilet your patient before sitting down to a meal.

- The short attention spans of Alzheimer patients can cause distraction. They are easily distracted by noises and activities around them. Whenever possible, eliminate noises created by the TV, radio, pets, and ringing telephones from the dining area.

- Restlessness during mealtime is also a problem. Consider playing soothing background music. It can have a calming effect on both you and your patient.

### What food-related distractions may cause mealtime problems?

- Some patients cannot cope with two different kinds of food consistencies on the same plate. For example, liquids and solids such as applesauce and vegetables may cause confusion. Pureeing the vegetables to match the consistency of the applesauce may help.

- Dishes with fancy patterns may be a source of visual confusion and distraction for your patient. Solid-color dishes contrasting with the color of the food being served may help.

- Offering an entire meal on a plate at the same time can be confusing and distracting. Try placing one food item at a time on the dish. Or use a separate plate for each food item. (Disposable plates save time and energy!)

- If you do place the entire meal on your patient's plate at one time, rotate the plate frequently. This will help your patient notice all the different foods on the plate.

- A diminished ability to taste different flavors may cause your patient to be distracted or uninterested in eating a meal if food has lost its appeal. Flavor enhancers can help. For example, chicken can be marinated with chicken broth to intensify taste and aroma. Strong flavors such as bacon and cheese added to soups and vegetables may also help.

## What eating-related problems will I encounter as physical and mental abilities decline? How can I help overcome these problems?

- Alzheimer patients develop visual difficulties. A strong contrast between the color of the plate and the food will allow the patient to see the food more easily. A solid-colored tablecloth that strongly contrasts with your dishes will also be helpful.

- Some patients forget how to use forks, knives, and spoons. They may begin to eat food with their fingers. If your patient has lost the ability to use eating utensils, consider new ways to make the food easier to hold. For example, offer French toast sticks instead of full slices for breakfast. For other meals, try using chicken sticks or nuggets instead of large pieces of chicken, or fish sticks in place of fish filets.

- Some patients experience tremors that may cause them to spill food frequently. Swivel spoons may be helpful. (See Appendix D)

- Plastic cups with sipping lids used for young children will help avoid spilled drinks.

- Some patients repeatedly drop food off their forks and spoons. To avoid food-soiled clothing, consider a washable, reusable adult-sized bib. (See Appendix D) Your patient may become upset at the prospect of wearing a bib. It may help if you are willing to set an example by also wearing one.

- Excessive drooling can be a problem. Try offering fruit nectar or juices in place of milk. Milk tends to promote drooling by increasing mucous production.

- Your patient may suddenly refuse to eat. This may be due to dental problems. Check for red or swollen gums or loose-fitting dentures. If your patient can still communicate, directly ask about mouth pain.

*What kind of chewing and swallowing problems may develop at mealtime? How can I solve these problems?*

- Some patients have trouble swallowing liquids. If your patient experiences this problem, thicken liquids with a thickening agent such as Thick N Easy by Hormel Foods. (See Appendix D) Or serve thickened liquids in the form of gelatins, puddings, yogurt, or ice cream.

- If your patient loves the taste of peanut butter but has a problem swallowing it, mix the peanut butter with applesauce for easier swallowing. Or, you can dilute the peanut butter in a blender with a small amount of water.

- Rough, crunchy-type foods such as raw carrots and celery, popcorn, or hard candies are often difficult to chew and swallow. If this becomes a problem, avoid giving these foods to your patient.

- If your patient has a mouthful of food but does not seem to be chewing, you may need to remind the patient to chew. Gently apply a light pressure with your hand under his or her chin and say, "Chew." A caution: if food is wedged in your patient's mouth, use a metal spoon to scoop it out. A plastic utensil may break if your patient clamps down on it. Try to avoid placing your fingers in your patient's mouth. You may get bitten.

- Some patients will chew endlessly. You simply have to remind them to swallow.

- Serve small portions of each item. By cutting foods into small pieces, chewing and swallowing will become easier.

*Are there certain foods or ways of serving foods that are dangerous to my patient?*

*YES! The following are important cautionary reminders to caregivers.*

- Keep your patient upright while eating. The patient's head should be tilted slightly forward. Never tilt his or her head back during eating. This precaution will help prevent accidental choking.

- Learn how to perform the Heimlich maneuver. It could save your patient's life. You will find step-by-step directions following this section for the Heimlich maneuver.

- Always check the temperature of foods or liquids before serving, especially if you use a microwave oven. Many Alzheimer patients have a reduced ability to feel pain. Or, they may not be able to verbalize that they are experiencing pain from overheated food.

- Be careful when serving large food objects. Make sure the food is cut into easily chewed sizes. An example would be hard-boiled eggs. Some patients may try to swallow an egg whole. Slice the egg before placing it on the table or near the patient.

- Avoid serving food items that have pits or bones. The patient may try to swallow them.

- Make sure you remove paper wrappings from foods. Patients have been known to swallow food wrappings.

- Keep soap and shaving cream or any other items that can be mistaken for food away from your patient.

- Don't place flowers in the eating area. Patients have been known to eat them.

- Keep your eye on napkins and paper cups during mealtime. Your patient may mistake them for food.

*Can I expect my patient to develop unusual food preferences?*

*Yes. The following are a few that your patient may experience. Here are some suggestions for dealing with them:*

- Some patients experience a diminished appetite. Offering smaller meals more frequently throughout the day may help insure that the patient is receiving proper nutrition. Try nutritional supplements such as Ensure if you are concerned about the nutritional value of your patient's food intake.

- Binge eating can become a problem. Alzheimer patients can develop all the same health-related maladies caused by excessive weight as any other individual. Monitor your patient's food intake throughout the day to be sure that you are aware of the accumulated amount of food he or she is consuming.

- A craving for sweets may develop, and some patients will eat tasty desserts before eating their meal. Be firm about limiting sweets until after the meal. Monitor your patient's daily intake of sweet snacks and desserts. Make sure these types of food do not interfere with the proper intake of nutritious foods.

- Some patients develop cravings for foods they once disliked. As long as your patient is receiving a balanced diet, these new cravings are not a problem unless they aggravate existing problems such as fluid retention.

*Can I expect my patient to develop unusual food-related behaviors?*

Yes, and some of these behaviors can endanger your patient.

- Some patients will hoard food. This behavior can be harmful since hidden food may become contaminated by the time a patient eats it. To avoid hoarding, try offering snacks throughout the day.

- Make sure that your patient is not removing food from trash containers in the home. Secure trash container lids whenever possible.

- As previously mentioned, patients will eat items that are not food. Perception and memory impairments are usually responsible for this behavior. Keep harmful objects and potentially poisonous medications and substances away from your patient's reach. Lock them away.

*What are the best times to feed my patient?*

- The best times are breakfast and lunchtime. As the day wears on, patients tend to fatigue. By dinnertime, some patients become irritable and uncooperative with efforts to feed them. If they have had adequate nutrition at breakfast and lunch, don't worry about dinnertime food intake.

*What can I do to make mealtime more pleasant?*

- Try serving five or six small meals a day instead of the traditional three main meals. Most Alzheimer patients eat sparingly because of appetite changes. They are more likely to accept a larger quantity of food per day with more frequent meal servings.

- Alzheimer patients function best when they have an established routine to follow. Try to serve meals at the same time each day. You may even want to announce each meal with some unique cue such as a chime or bell.

- Make an effort to have your patient eat in the presence of other people. For many, mealtime means a time to be with others. Eating in a family or social setting allows Alzheimer patients to continue this important ritual.

*How can I make mealtime less difficult and irritating?*

- Most Alzheimer patients take longer to eat than other people. Plan to allow extra time for meals.

- Don't worry about poor table manners. It is an exercise in futility to try to educate someone who can no longer learn. What they eat is more important than how they eat.

- If you are dining out with an Alzheimer patient, carry a special card that reads: "My companion has Alzheimer's disease and may not understand you. Please direct questions to me." Give this card to the wait staff before someone comes to take your order. Reassure the staff that you will manage any problems that may arise.

### How can I make serving food less troublesome for my patient?

- When serving from closed containers, remember to remove the lids. If your patient can't see the food inside, he or she may not realize that food is under the lid.

- Try placing a damp washcloth under the plate to reduce sliding of your patient's dish. Rubberized materials used to line shelves and drawers also work well when placed under dishes to keep them from sliding. Special plates are also available with suction cups that hold the plate to the table. (See Appendix D)

- To prevent liquid spills, use cups with lids that hold securely. Cups are available with container lids with a hole in which to place a straw. (See Appendix D)

- The use of straws is ideal for a patient with advanced dementia since many of these patients forget how to drink from a cup. But they retain the ability to suck liquid through a straw.

- Some patients cannot swallow cereal served with milk. They tend to prefer dry cereal. For these patients, serve the milk separately.

- If your patient tells you that food "tastes strange," he or she may be trying to say that the food has little or no flavor. A note of caution: Patients with decaying teeth or those who drink too much alcohol have been known to say that food "tastes strange." Try to determine the cause of your patient's complaint about the taste of food. Marinating meat, fish, or poultry in salad dressings, soups, gravies, or even fruit juices will enhance their flavors. You may also try using strong herbs for flavoring such as basil, oregano, or rosemary.

- Some patients will not drink milk if they do not see it poured into the cup from the container. If this happens, be sure your patient sees you pouring the milk into the cup.

- Offer only one kind of eating utensil if your patient seems to have forgotten how to use different utensils or becomes confused when offered more than one kind at a time.

*Are there nutritional concerns about my patient's diet? What can I do?*

- Dehydration is always a concern with Alzheimer patients. Pay attention to fluid intake, especially if your patient has been vomiting or has had diarrhea. Ask your family physician about the amount of fluids your patient should drink daily. (See Dehydration in Chapter 2.)

- If you have difficulty getting your patient to eat a balanced diet, ask your physician about vitamin supplements or if liquid nutritional drinks would be appropriate.

- Try to "punch up" the nutrition of some foods. A few suggestions are: add wheat germ to soups or shredded carrots to tuna fish. Try sprinkling grated lemon rind on fruit or vegetable salads. Use your imagination. If your patient doesn't like your experiment, go back to the original dish and try something else.

# The Heimlich Maneuver
## When and How to Use It On a Conscious Choking Victim

**(This information is not intended as a substitute for
professional medical advice or treatment.)**

You know your own patient's communicative abilities best. If your patient is either uncooperative or cannot respond to directions, you should call 911 immediately if he or she appears to be choking, especially if someone else is present to begin the Heimlich maneuver while you make the call. Otherwise, immediately begin performing the Heimlich maneuver as soon as you've called 911.

Generally, a 911 call is placed after it becomes obvious that the Heimlich maneuver is not working. But since Alzheimer patients have a diminished ability to communicate, you do not want to waste precious time. Emergency medical personnel would rather respond to an unneeded call than to lose a patient because they arrived late.

*When should I perform the Heimlich maneuver?*
Perform the Heimlich maneuver **immediately** if your patient is conscious, looks alarmed, and:

- Is not breathing

- Is clutching his or her throat

- Is choking, but is not coughing

- Displays a weak or ineffective cough. This indicates that air exchange is minimal and that you should start the Heimlich maneuver.

- Is unable to speak (if he or she is still normally capable of speaking)

- Has a bluish appearance to his or her skin color

*How do I perform the Heimlich maneuver?*
**(NOTE: You should practice this technique before you may need to perform it.)**

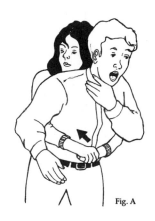

1. If seated, help your patient to stand up. If your patient is much larger than you, leave the patient seated. If possible, turn the patient sideways in the chair so that his or her back is exposed to you.

2. Place yourself slightly behind your patient. (Fig. A)

3. Place your arms around your patient's waist.

Fig. A

4. Make a fist with one hand with your thumb toward your patient. Place your fist just above his or her belly button.

5. Grab your fist with your other hand.

6. Deliver five upward squeeze-thrusts into the patient's abdomen.

7. Make each squeeze-thrust strong enough to dislodge a foreign body from your patient's airway.

*What should happen next?*

- Your thrusts will make the diaphragm move air out of the patient's lungs. It should create an artificial cough.

- Keep a firm grip on your patient. If the Heimlich maneuver has not been effective, your patient could lose consciousness and fall down.

- Repeat the Heimlich maneuver until the foreign body is expelled.

- If your patient cannot expel the foreign body after repeated tries, call 911 for help if you haven't already done so.

*How should I perform the Heimlich maneuver if my patient is conscious but lying down?*

- Turn your patient face up and tilt his chin slightly upward. (Fig. B)

- Position yourself over his body. Then place both of your hands at the bottom of the patient's belly (just above the belly button) and perform the upward thrusts as shown to dislodge the foreign object. (Fig. C) This forces air up through the throat and causes the food to pop out.

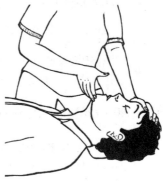

Fig. B

*Are there special precautions I should take with the Heimlich maneuver?*

- To avoid breaking your patient's bones, <u>never</u> place your hands on his or her breastbone or lower rib cage when performing the Heimlich maneuver.

Fig. C

# Bathing, Oral Hygiene, and Grooming

Bathing presents problems that involve both safety and emotional issues. Although bathing is something they've done since birth, it can become a frightening experience for Alzheimer patients. Many of the aspects of bathing that they once took for granted may seem strange and create fear in your patient. For example, the sudden sensation of water against their skin can startle some Alzheimer patients, or even be mistaken as an assault.

Good oral hygiene plays an important role in the health of your patient. Mouth infections, sore gums, and pain from cavities or ill-fitting dentures may cause your patient to avoid eating, which can lead to nutritional deficiencies.

Personal grooming such as hair care, shaving, make-up and nail care needs monitoring. If your patient is capable of taking care of these daily needs, allow the patient to do as much as he or she can safely do. But don't hesitate to assist whenever you believe that time has come.

Since a strong sense of independence can cause an Alzheimer patient to rail against help with daily hygiene and grooming, these important activities can become a challenge. The following suggestions will help you and your patient overcome this challenge.

### When is the best time of day to bathe an Alzheimer patient?

- Changing old habits can generate frustration and anger. If your patient has had the life-long habit of bathing in the morning or evening, don't try to change their routine.

### How can I avoid arguments when trying to bathe my patient?

- If you encounter resistance to the bathing process, try convincing your patient to agree to one small step in the process at a time. For example, say, "Okay, we'll bathe later. Let's take your shoes off now." Then go on to the next step.

- Giving your patient a sense of control may also help. Say, "When would you like to take a bath?" Or ask the patient, "How about if we bathe in about ten minutes." Let your patient know that you respect his or her decision, but that bathing must be done.

- On occasion, if your patient steadfastly refuses to bathe and becomes highly agitated, consider whether it is better to skip a bath that time. A brief cleansing at the bathroom basin may be an alternative now and again.

- It is also helpful to break up the bathing care routine into a series of small steps. One approach may be to say, "First, let's take the washcloth and wash your face." (This approach is useful in other areas of personal hygiene as well, such as tooth brushing.)

*What else can I do to make the bathing routine more pleasant?*

- Ask your patient whether the bathroom feels warm enough. If the bathroom feels cold to the patient, consider using an additional heater in the area. *Caution: make sure the patient is safely away from the heater at all times. Keep the heater away from water.*

- Placing a seat in the shower area may lessen the resistance of a patient to taking a shower. Plastic molded shower chairs are available in many home health stores.

- Bubble baths help some patients to enjoy and even look forward to bathing.

- If you encounter real resistance to a bathing routine, try a reward system. In return for the patient's cooperation, offer him or her the opportunity for extra television watching, or an extra visit from a family member. You may want to offer a candy bar as a reward since some Alzheimer patients have an abnormal craving for sweets.

*What if I cannot convince my patient to cooperate with the bathing routine?*

- If a patient refuses to enter a tub or shower, try a sponge bath at the bathroom basin.

- If you or someone in the household is comfortable bathing with the patient, that may be the answer. Often, it is reassuring to the patient to not be alone in the tub or shower. Your patient may welcome bathing as a fun activity.

- If your patient complains about shampoo burning his or her eyes, use tearless baby shampoo for hair washing.

*How can I help my patient if he or she is fearful of entering a shower?*

- Sometimes this fear can be overcome by adjusting the water temperature first. Let the patient feel the water with his or her hands before stepping into the shower.

- A spray nozzle that delivers a very fine spray may help. Some Alzheimer patients have sensitive skin and find the normal pressure of a showerhead objectionable.

*How much freedom should I allow my patient during the bathing routine?*

- Allow your patient to do as much of the bathing procedure as he or she can safely do without help. Some Alzheimer patients retain a strong sense of independence, and prefer to do as much as possible for themselves. It is extremely important to allow your patient to feel some sense of control however small or bothersome it may seem to you.

*What safety precautions should I take with the bathing routine?*

- While in the shower or tub, Alzheimer patients should not stand on one leg at any time. Many patients have impaired balance. Standing on one leg could markedly increase their risk of falling.

- Privacy is important to respect, but safety is always an overriding factor with Alzheimer patients. Someone should always be in the bathroom with the patient, even if he or she is in the shower or tub alone.

- It is best to use a shower chair with a built-in back support. But if your patient is sitting in a shower chair without a back support, try providing support for the patient's back or shoulder blades with your hand.

*What problems may I encounter while helping my patient with oral hygiene? How can I deal with these problems?*

- Make sure your patient is keeping up with oral hygiene. A patient who is still capable of other forms of personal hygiene may be neglecting that important function. Check your patient's mouth at bath time or after each meal.

- If your patient uses dentures, examine his or her mouth frequently for any signs of pain or gum irritation. These problems can result in poor nutrition if you patient is hesitant to chew food properly.

- Remember the caution from "Dealing with Mealtime Problems." Avoid putting your fingers into your patient's mouth, if possible. You don't want to get bitten. And when removing built-up food particles from your patient's mouth, use metal utensils or instruments instead of plastic.

- Tooth or denture cleaning requires a complex sequence of tasks. Your patient may lose the memory of part of that routine, which can result in poor oral hygiene and its related consequences.

  *A hint: line the bathroom sink with a washcloth to avoid breaking dentures if they are dropped.*

- You can observe whether your patient is missing a part of the procedure by breaking down the steps of tooth or denture cleaning for him or her.

- Don't hesitate to consult your dentist about proper tooth cleaning. The dentist may also have helpful tips for you to help make oral hygiene more effective and less frustrating.

- Some patients may resist your help with oral hygiene. They may perceive your help as an intrusion into an intimate part of their body. The patient may actually clench his or her teeth. Patience and gentleness can help overcome this behavior. But you can clean clenched teeth from the outside if it becomes necessary.

- Soft bristled toothbrushes may help a tender mouth. Also, sponges embedded with toothpaste and attached to sticks are available at some drugstores.

*What personal grooming issues will need my attention?*

For the health and self-esteem of your patient, personal grooming such as hair care, shaving, make-up, and nail care should continue even after your patient can no longer assist you.

*How can I make hair care as easy as possible?*

- Keep the hair cut in an easy-to-manage length and style.

- Use the kitchen sink to wash your patient's hair if that is easier than the bathtub or shower. Buy a hose/spray attachment for easy rinsing.

- Find a hair stylist or barber willing to make house calls. Even if your patient is comfortable in a salon or barbershop, prepare ahead for when that is no longer true.

*What about shaving for male patients and applying make-up for female patients?*

- For male patients – supervise shaving until it becomes too difficult. Later, an electric razor may make shaving easier and safer for both of you.

- For female patients – if your patient has always worn make-up and feels more comfortable wearing it, continue to help her feel good about herself. You can tone down the process to lipstick and powder. Eye make-up is too hard to apply to someone else and allowing the patient to apply eye make-up herself may result in an eye injury.

  *Note: Alzheimer patients may be frightened by their reflection in a mirror and not recognize themselves. If this occurs, keep the mirror covered when your patient is present in a room.*

## *What about nail care?*

- When your patient can no longer safely trim fingernails and toenails, begin to take over the chore.

- Trim nails about twice a month. If your patient is uncooperative during trimmings, allow him or her to watch television or listen to music during that time.

- A visit to a podiatrist once every 3–6 months may be helpful, especially if your patient has difficulty with toenails, bunions, or calluses.

# Toileting and Bathroom Needs

At a very early age, we learn that getting rid of bodily wastes in the proper way is an important part of being "grown up." We also learn that it is a very private function. Therefore the loss of bladder and bowel control that comes with Alzheimer's can be an affront to the dignity of the patient.

As a caregiver, keeping a patient clean and dry along with the safety issues around toileting often take precedence over the concerns of how the patient is feeling about this powerfully emotional situation. Finding a balance between the patient's dignity and the caregiver's daily duties can be accomplished.

The following suggest how to handle problems with toileting and incontinence as they arise:

### How can I help make trips to the bathroom safe?

- Consider installing nightlights in a hallway leading to the bathroom.

- Install grab bars near the toilet. Grab bars can be purchased in home building supply stores and home health catalogs.

- If the bathroom doorknob can be locked, make sure you have a key close by in case your patient becomes locked in. Practice unlocking the door before you need to in a hurry.

### What can I do to make bathroom use less frustrating?

- Many Alzheimer patients have very poor vision. Placing a sign on the bathroom door identifying that room may prove helpful. Placing an enlarged photo of a toilet near the sign could prove even more helpful.

- Develop a routine bathroom schedule for your patient. Keeping a diary of your patient's toileting habits will give you a clue to how frequently a trip to the bathroom is necessary. Until you establish a pattern, a suggested schedule might be every two hours. Scheduling helps the patient develop a routine of regular trips to the bathroom.

- Try to respect your patient's privacy by closing the bathroom door if others are in the area. Keep the door slightly ajar to allow for quick access, if necessary.

- Some patients evacuate their bowels very slowly because of immobility. Giving the patient a magazine to look at while he or she is on the toilet may prevent the patient from becoming restless.

*How do I know if my patient needs to use the bathroom if he or she does not tell me?*

- If the patient displays restlessness and begins to pull at his or her clothing, this behavior may be a sign that it is time for a visit to the bathroom.

- Be aware that the consumption of alcohol or caffeine by your patient will increase the need to urinate more frequently.

- Caffeine consumption in the morning may also result in a need to move the bowels.

*How should I decide if incontinence pads/pants (adult diapers) are appropriate for my patient?*

- The decision to use adult diapers can only be made by the individual caregiver. Some caregivers believe that the use of diapers will be an insult to their patient's dignity. However, the patient may actually feel more secure wearing a diaper rather than constantly worrying about his or her bowel and bladder function and the embarrassment of an "accident."

*If I am having trouble keeping adult diapers in place, what can I do?*

- If the diaper won't stay on, try cutting the legs away from a pair of pantyhose. Place the panty section of the hose over the diaper to hold it in place.

*Are there any remedies I can use to protect my patient's skin in the diaper area?*

- Check the skin around the diaper area and change the diaper as soon as it is wet.

- Sprinkle cornstarch around the groin area to help maintain dryness. Place the cornstarch inside a clean sock or knee-hi pantyhose stocking. Secure the top with a rubber band. Sprinkle by gently tapping the sock or stocking around the groin area. *Note: Don't overdo – cornstarch can clump on the patient's skin.*

- Use protective lotions such as A & D Ointment or Vaseline to help prevent serious skin problems.

- Be careful not to get plastic diaper tabs stuck to the skin. If your patient's skin is sensitive, it may cause skin irritation.

# Coping With Sleeping Problems

Many Alzheimer patients have disturbed sleep. Studies show that these patients spend less time in both deep and dreaming states of sleep. In addition, the 24-hour sleep-wake cycle is disturbed. This alteration causes Alzheimer patients to sleep more during the day and to stay awake longer at night.

Alzheimer patients may experience sleep disturbances for other reasons as well. The following discussion will explain a few and offer solutions.

*What are some other reasons Alzheimer patients have trouble sleeping? How can I help my patient sleep better?*

- Illness or pain may keep a patient awake. If sleep disturbance is ongoing, it would be wise to take your patient for a medical checkup.

- Depression can cause trouble with falling asleep. If you suspect that your patient is depressed, a physician should assess the situation. If depression is the problem, your physician may prescribe an antidepressant-sedative to help.

- Caffeine, a stimulant found in many soft drinks, tea, and coffee, may keep the patient from sleeping well. Reduce or eliminate caffeine intake by using decaffeinated drinks.

- Hunger may keep a patient awake at night. A bedtime snack such as warm milk is helpful. Remember that hot cocoa contains chocolate, which may act as a stimulant.

- Lack of physical exercise, such as walking during the day, may create sleeping problems for patients who are more active at night.

*What about the use of over-the-counter medications for sleeping problems?*

- You should always check with your physician before giving Alzheimer patients any medications.

*Are there ways to make my patient's bedroom more conducive to sleep?*

- The bedroom may feel too hot or too cold. Ask your patient if the room temperature feels okay.

- Some patients become disoriented if a sleeping room is totally darkened. If that's true for your patient, consider using several nightlights placed throughout the room.

- Some patients are afraid of the dark. For these patients, in addition to a nightlight, a softly playing radio may help alleviate their fear of the dark.

- Try using the gradual dimming of lights (with a dimmer switch) as a cue to announce sleep time.

### How can I make the bed and bedding more comfortable for my patient?

- Use quilts instead of blankets. Quilts are less likely to tangle than blankets.

- Allow your patient to use a favorite quilt and pillow. If hospitalized, send this favorite bedding with your patient if the hospital will grant your request.

- Bed rails should be used cautiously. They may successfully restrain some patients. However, other patients may try to climb over the bed rails resulting in injury.

- Place your patient's bed against the wall, if possible. That will eliminate at least one area of the bed as potentially dangerous for falls.

# Coping With Sundowning

Sundowning refers to a pattern of behavior in some Alzheimer patients. The name refers to changes in the patient as the sun goes down. These patients are relatively energetic during the early part of the day but by day's end, they become tired and more cognitively impaired. Some may become restless and agitated. Often, sundown behavior becomes apparent at dinnertime.

*What causes sundowning in some patients?*
- Certain cardiovascular conditions
- Polypharmacy (the taking of too many drugs at one time)
- Low intake of water by the patient

*Are there some outdoor daytime activities that can help lessen the effects of sundowning?*

- Studies have shown that daily exposure to daylight is the single best way to normalize sundowning in Alzheimer patients.

- If possible, expose your patient to some gentle outdoor activity each day such as taking a walk. Remember to include periodic rest breaks.
  *Note: In planning exercise for your patient, it is extremely important to check with your patient's physician. Make sure there are no underlying medical problems that would prohibit exercise.*

*What can I do inside the home to help avoid sundowning?*

- Play quiet music in the late afternoon in place of a loud radio or television.

- Turn lights on inside your home long before it gets dark outside. This will help adjust your patient to the end of the day.

- Don't allow your patient to rest in a dark room during the day. He or she may awaken and think it is early morning.

- Have your patient take daytime naps while sitting upright in a chair – not reclined on a bed. When a patient awakens in bed, he or she tends to think it is a new day.

## Chapter Topics and Suggested Readings
## from the Alzheimer's Association 2001 Public Publications Catalog:

(See Introduction [pg. ii] to learn how to receive these publications.)

Meeting Daily Challenges – VHS video – covers most topics in this chapter.

### Dealing with Mealtime Problems
Eating – fact sheet
Nutrition – fact sheet

### Bathing, Oral Hygiene, and Personal Grooming
Steps to Assisting with Personal Care: Overcoming Challenges and Adapting to the
Needs of Persons with Alzheimer's Disease – brochure
Bathing – fact sheet
Dental Care – fact sheet
Dressing – fact sheet

### Coping with Sundowning
Shadowing and Sundowning – fact sheet

# Chapter Two

## Handling Common
## Medical Problems

*~ " The true test of character is not how much we know how to do,
but how we behave when we don't know what to do" ~*

John Holt

# *Administering Medications*

Alzheimer patients experience problems that make swallowing medications difficult. Here are a few suggestions to make this important chore less difficult for the patient and the caregiver.

### *Is it okay to break a pill into smaller pieces for my patient?*

- *Caution: Some medicines should only be taken whole.* Please check with your pharmacist before breaking pills or tablets for your patient.

- In general, if a pill or tablet has a score line down the center, it can be made smaller or crushed without a problem.

- A bitter taste may be present in cut or crushed pills. If this is a problem for your patient, disguise the taste by placing the pill in peanut butter, gelatin, applesauce, pudding, etc.

### *Are there other ways to make a pill easier for my patient to swallow?*

- Pills that cannot or should not be crushed or medication in capsule form can be coated with butter to make them easier to swallow.

### *What if my patient cannot swallow medications due to dry mouth?*

- Have your patient drink some water. Tell your patient to swish some of the water around in his or her mouth before you administer the medication.

- Before giving medications to a patient with dry mouth, have the patient try to chew gum or suck on soft candy to stimulate saliva flow.
  *Note: Use extreme caution. Don't place hard candy in a patient's mouth if he or she is so impaired that the candy may possibly be swallowed whole.*

### *Are there any foods that I can mix medications with before giving them to my patient?*

- Try mixing pills in applesauce, apple butter, or maple syrup, or any food your patient likes and can safely swallow.

- Mix a small amount of food with whole or crushed pills. Follow with a spoonful of the same food.

### *What if I'm having trouble getting my patient to swallow many pills each day?*

- Place priority on the most important pills. For example, if your patient is taking a cardiac pill and a stool softener, make sure the patient gets the cardiac pill on time. The stool softener can be given past its usual time of administration.

Always check with your physician regarding which medications are of the utmost importance for your patient.

# Constipation

Alzheimer patients may not recognize that they are constipated. They may feel discomfort but not associate it with constipation. You will need to keep a check on your patient's frequency of bowel movements.

Constipation has many causes. The most serious complication is a bowel obstruction. Constipation remedies can do more harm than good if there is an obstruction. So, if constipation is prolonged and not relieved with simple remedies or by laxatives and Fleet enemas, have your patient checked by a physician for a possible bowel obstruction.

### What are some of the signs and symptoms of constipation?

- Hard, dry stools

- Lower than normal number of stools

- Straining during a bowel movement

If your patient complains of abdominal discomfort or if you notice abdominal distension (extra fullness), inform your physician.

### What are some other causes of constipation among Alzheimer patients?

- A diet low in fiber. A lesser-known contributing factor to constipation is loss of teeth. The loss of teeth among some elderly people results in the eating of soft processed foods, which often lack fiber. Dietary fiber is needed to help avoid constipation.

- A diet high in fats (too much meat, eggs, and dairy products).

- Prolonged bed rest.

- An underactive thyroid gland.

- Loss of body fluids due to prolonged nausea or vomiting.

- Insufficient water intake.

### How can I help my patient avoid or reduce the frequency of constipation?

- Establish a regular toileting schedule.

- Encourage more fluid intake – ask your physician to determine what is proper for the patient. Try serving different kinds of fluids. For example, offer a glass of fruit juice and a glass of milk. Both are fluids that will help relieve constipation. Pulpy fruit juices are especially good since they contain fiber.

- Check with your pharmacist or family physician about the side effects of your patient's medications. Some drugs can cause constipation. Taking several medications, all with constipation as a side effect, will increase the problem. Ask your physician if it is safe to increase your patient's daily fluid intake if your patient is taking medications with constipation as a side effect.

- Develop a regular exercise program, which can help reduce constipation. Many Alzheimer patients retain the ability to walk for a very long time. (Studies have shown that regular walking programs also increase thinking and memory abilities and decrease depression and anxiety in Alzheimer patients. But these effects last only as long as exercise is maintained.) Check with your physician for any restrictions to exercising.

### *What remedies can I offer my patient to relieve constipation?*

- Serve your patient applesauce at least three times daily.

- Each morning, serve your patient lightly warmed prune juice.

- The following formula was reported to be very effective for constipation by R. Behm in the 1985 issue of *Geriatric Nursing*: Mix 1 cup applesauce, 1 cup unprocessed bran, and 1/2 cup of pure prune juice. Take 1 or 2 tablespoons of the mix at bedtime.

- Bulk-forming additives such as bran and psyllium-containing products.

- If the above remedies are not effective, try a Fleet's enema (not a standard, full-size enema), milk of magnesia, or glycerin suppositories.

- Try stool softeners, but they are better as a preventative to constipation.

### *Should I check with my physician before using some over-the-counter remedies for my patient?*

Yes. Check with your physician before using the following remedies for relief.

- Dulcolax suppositories. (Use one each morning for a few weeks. These usually work within 10 to 20 minutes but can work any time after insertion. It may be best to use after breakfast to avoid mealtime interruption for a bathroom break.)

- Dulcolax in pill form.

- Full-sized enemas.

# Dehydration

Dehydration is a serious loss of body water. Alzheimer patients, especially those in institutions and those in the later stages of the disease, are prone to dehydration. The reason for this problem is not clear, but it may be related to the disease process.

When Alzheimer patients were experimentally dehydrated, it was found that they didn't feel the need to drink as do people without the disease.

Sometimes, Alzheimer patients simply forget to drink water. If your patient has diabetes or has had diarrhea and or vomiting, it is crucial that you make sure he or she drinks sufficient amounts of water or fluids.

(Note: Some solid foods count as liquid intake, for example: gelatin, sherbets and ice cream, and any food that turns to liquid at room temperature.)

### *How can I help my patient avoid dehydration?*

- Set up a regular drinking schedule for your patient.  Some authorities say that every 2 to 3 hours is best. Others have suggested offering fluids every half hour.  Try to strike a happy medium with your patient between these two suggestions.

- Many Alzheimer patients fear losing urinary control, so they may try to avoid fluid intake. Keep your patient on a regular toileting schedule to help reduce this fear. Reassure your patient that you will help him or her to the bathroom and that you will clean up wetting accidents if they occur.

## Urinary Incontinence

Urinary incontinence is caused by many factors in Alzheimer patients such as infection or stress. Prostate problems in men and leaking due to weakening of the muscles in the bladders of women can cause urinary incontinence. Some medications such as diuretics also can cause excess urine excretion.

It is important to the patient's emotional well being that you don't make a big issue of an incident of incontinence. Patients are not deliberately incontinent and may become very embarrassed and feel ashamed when an episode occurs.

Keeping your incontinent patient's skin dry is essential because wet clothing can very quickly lead to skin irritations, rashes, and sores that will be difficult to heal.

*Are there reasons for incontinence not medically related? What can I do to help?*

Some incontinence problems relate to the patient's diminished mental capacity. But there are ways to work around these problems.

- Incontinence can occur simply because your patient can't find the bathroom. Try lighting hallways that lead to the bathroom. You may also find that placing large-sized signs and a picture of a toilet near the bathroom to be helpful.

- Finding the toilet can be a problem. Changing the toilet seat color to one that contrasts with the floor may be helpful.

- Limited mobility may contribute to incontinence if a patient cannot reach the bathroom in time. For these patients, you may want to provide a bedroom commode.

- If your patient is taking a diuretic, be ready for it to work quickly and often. Try to give the diuretic first thing in the morning. The effects of the diuretic will then taper off throughout the day.

- Patients may become incontinent because they won't void if they are not provided enough privacy. Try to provide that needed privacy whenever possible. A suggestion would be to use a foldable, movable screen on wheels.

- Some patients become incontinent because they cannot undress themselves quickly enough. Garment modification may help this problem. Garments with elastic waistbands such as jogging pants and wraparound skirts work well. Flap-type underwear may also be useful.

- Some patients are unable to express or sense an urgency to urinate. Placing your patient on a routine toileting schedule will help. A suggested time schedule would be approximately every two hours.

*What can I do about nighttime incontinence?*

- Avoid excess fluid intake before bedtime.

- Place the bed low to the floor (if your patient can comfortably get out of the bed in that position) and near the bathroom or commode.

- Place a waterproof protector over the mattress. Cover it with a fitted bottom sheet and tuck it in securely. *Note: A mattress protector may cause some patients to sweat excessively; discontinue use if this happens.*

*How can I make my incontinent patient more comfortable?*

- Try pull-up type adult diapers. Check the fit. If your patient is a heavy wetter, use thick, heavily padded diapers. Some contain a fluid-absorbing gel that helps keep the patient drier than other types.

- If your patient has a wet diaper and is sitting down, don't try to pull the diaper from under the patient while he or she is still sitting. Lift your patient up and then pull out the diaper. Skin breakdown can occur if you pull too hard on the diaper if it pulls against the skin. If necessary, cut the sides of the diaper. If the diaper is dry, you can tape it back together.

  *Note: Be careful not to get adhesive tape stuck to your patient's skin.*

- To prevent skin irritation from wet diapers, first dry the area and then apply an ointment such as Desitin or other diaper rash ointments, or petroleum jelly. These products help create a barrier against wetness on the patient's skin.

- Always check the skin around the buttocks and genitals for skin redness, which is an initial sign of irritation that leads to skin infection or ulceration. Keep all areas dry and clean. A little extra time spent in prevention can save major skin problems later.

  *(See Chapter 1, Helping Your Patient with Toileting and Bathroom Needs for additional tips)*

# Urinary Tract Infections

Urinary tract infections are relatively common in Alzheimer patients. These patients generally eat poorly and the resultant malnutrition weakens their immune systems making them susceptible to urinary tract infections.

*How will I know if my patient has a urinary tract infection?*

- If your patient is still able to communicate, he or she may tell you that urinating stings and causes discomfort.

*What should I look for if my patient no longer communicates verbally?*

- Urine that is dark or cloudy in color, or contains blood.

- Urine that smells particularly pungent.

- A reduction in the frequency of urination and the passing of smaller amounts.

*How can I help avoid or decrease the incidence of urinary tract infections for my patient?*

- Get your patient out of bed and moving as much as possible. Urinary tract infections are more common in patients with prolonged bed rest.

- If your patient is confined to bed, consult a physical therapist about the proper way to perform passive motion exercises on your patient.

- Encourage your patient to drink plenty of water. Urinary tract infections are more common among those who are dehydrated.

- Serve cranberry juice or vitamin C to make the urine more acidic. Acidic urine tends to inhibit bacteria. ***Check with your physician first before offering acidic fluids to your patient.***

# Skin Ulcers

Skin ulcers are common in bedridden Alzheimer patients. Immobility increases the risk for the formation of ulcers because circulation is poor. Ill-fitting clothing and malnutrition also can contribute to ulcer formation. Since Alzheimer patients do not or cannot communicate effectively, a developing skin ulcer can go undetected. Check your patient carefully each day for any signs of skin ulcers.

Skin ulcers are more likely to occur over bony prominences. The weight of the body reduces blood supply to skin tissue. Fatty cushions over bony prominences can help prevent ulcer formation.

### Are there any strategies to build up fat reserves if my patient is undernourished or malnourished?

- One strategy would be to serve whole, fatted milk. You can also give your patient peanut butter, cheese, ice cream, or chocolate milk.

- For patients with heart problems, the above-mentioned food items might normally need to be restricted. But in a patient with severe malnutrition, the heart factor may be of lesser immediate concern. *Check with your physician about dietary changes for your patient if heart problems are present.*

- Malnourished patients should have daily multi-vitamin supplements containing zinc. The multi-vitamin will help ensure that your patient's minimum basic requirements are being met. Zinc tends to speed wound healing.

### What else can I do to help my patient avoid skin ulcers?

- If your patient is bedridden, try to change his or her position frequently at regularly scheduled intervals such as every few hours.

- Place padding under bony prominences. Avoid the use of rough towels. Towels can be wrapped in soft pillowcases.

- Urine can severely burn surrounding tissue. It is essential to clean and dry these areas quickly. To treat skin areas that are wet with urine, wash and clean the area with water and a good soap containing moisturizing lotion. Applying ointment such as a hydrocortisone cream may also help. *Check with your physician about the frequency with which you can safely use hydrocortisone creams.*

- Skin that displays redness, indentation, or where pronounced heat can be felt needs special treatment. A sterile dressing with antibiotic ointment is NOT the treatment of choice. This type of skin ulcer should be evaluated by a healthcare professional.

### What are the signs and symptoms of skin infection?

The acronym STAR will help you remember: Swelling, Tenderness, And, Redness.

*Chapter Topics and Suggested Readings*
*from the Alzheimer's Association 2001 Public Publications Catalog:*

**Administering Medications**
Medications – fact sheet


**Urinary Incontinence**
Incontinence – fact sheet

# Chapter Three

## Dealing With Mental
## And
## Emotional Decline

~ *"If you are patient in one moment of anger, you will escape a hundred days of sorrow"* ~

Chinese Proverb

# Communicating

As the process of dementia progresses, communication will become increasingly frustrating. Your patient may lose the ability to process complex sentences or instructions. The ability to speak or articulate effectively is also lost. When these problems are combined with the anger and aggressiveness Alzheimer patients sometimes exhibit, communicating can become a difficult challenge.

You can meet this challenge and soften its impact on your daily patterns of communication. Listen to your patient. Become aware of the subtle, or not so subtle, changes in your patient's ability or willingness to interact with you. Employing the following techniques as your patient's needs continually change will help.

### How can I communicate questions to my patient more effectively?

- Ask only one question at a time.

- Don't ask complex questions. Phrase questions so they may be answered with a simple "yes" or "no."

- If your patient does not answer your question, repeat the question slowly using *exactly* the same words. Keep your tone even to avoid showing frustration in your voice.

### How can I simplify communicating?

- Don't give your patient too many choices. Using a statement rather than a question may eliminate some communication problems. For example: say, "It is time to shower" instead of "Would you like to shower?"

- When asking your patient a question, allow more time for an answer than you ordinarily would. Alzheimer patients need more time to collect their thoughts and express their desires.

- Speak slowly. If your patient is hard of hearing, use a slightly louder tone of voice.

- Speak calmly, using low-pitched voice sounds. High-pitched sounds may be interpreted as anger by your patient. Many older people lose the ability to hear high-pitched sounds. This problem is more pronounced in Alzheimer patients.

- Always address the patient face to face at an equal height level. If your patient is sitting, you should also sit. To foster better communication, it is important psychologically to your patient that he or she is on equal footing with you.

- If it becomes obvious to you that your patient cannot find the right word to respond with, you might suggest the word you think the patient means. Confirm your word choice by saying, "Is this what you mean?" or "Is that the word your were looking for?"

- Don't use pronouns such as he, she, or it. They are too abstract for an Alzheimer patient to grasp. Use specific nouns and names such as John, Mary, the dog, etc. in place of pronouns.

### What are the most effective ways to ask my patient to perform a task or respond to a request?

- Keep your sentences as short as possible, preferably no more than five or six words in length.

- Break down the sequence of tasks into steps. For example, placing clothing on the bed in the order in which they should be put on will help when you verbalize each step involved in getting dressed.

- Be consistent with word choices. Always use the same word to describe the same thing. For example, if you use the word "toilet," continue to use "toilet." Don't change the word from toilet to other words such as bathroom or john.

- Avoid controlling language; it implies superiority on your part. Your patient may resent the request you are making because of your word choice, not because of the requested task itself. For example, your patient will perceive "John, lunch is here. Come eat your lunch now." as more demanding than "John, your lunch is ready."

### If my patient does not respond to my efforts to communicate, could there be other reasons for this lack of response?

If a patient is not communicating well, there may be several contributing factors. Any of the following may cause your patient to withdraw verbally:

- Too much background noise

- Too many people crowding around your patient

- A sudden change in daily routine

- Exhaustion - your patient may be physically tired

### If my patient has lost the ability to speak, are there other ways to communicate?

As patients lose their ability to speak in later stages of dementia, both you and your patient must learn to rely more on body language. For example, you can often read feelings from eye expression. This is particularly true for signs of physical pain and/or discomfort.

- If your patient exhibits negative behavior such as stealing food, try to focus on why that happened rather than on the act of stealing. Perhaps your patient is simply hungry and needs more to eat.

- Patients who have lost the ability to speak may respond favorably to a smile or to being gently touched.

# Managing Anger and Aggression

Alzheimer patients can become angry, anxious, and/or aggressive. As in dealing with other aspects of Alzheimer's, it is essential that you become alert to the subtle and overt changes that occur in your loved one's emotional behavior. Although there is often little time for constant vigilance of every nuance of your patient's mood, sometimes that is the most effective way to solve a small problem before it becomes a big one.

Some common situations that may precipitate angry or aggressive behavior are patient fatigue, travel, or sudden changes in routine. As Alzheimer's progresses, patients lose the ability to process stimuli. Too much background noise can be overwhelming. Excessive noise or sensory stimulation such as you find on many television programs can also irritate an Alzheimer patient. Avoid crowded public places if sensory overload is a problem. The following techniques will help you manage or minimize negative behaviors.

***Where is sensory overload most likely to happen? How can I avoid sensory overload for my patient?***

- Busy restaurants or shopping malls may increase confusion and cause sensory overload. Avoid taking your patient to malls, if possible. Shop at smaller, less-congested stores when your patient is with you.

- Buzzers or doorbells can create anxiety. Voices coming from overhead pagers or speakers can cause suspicion, confusion, and even paranoia in some cases.

- Religious services may be so crowded that they cause increased anxiety. Attend either very early or very late religious services if they are usually less crowded.

***Could undetected pain cause my patient to suddenly become angry or aggressive?***

Yes, pain can cause an Alzheimer patient to become angry. Some patients are unable to tell you that they are in pain. You may have to do a little detective work to find the origin of their pain. For example:

- One possible cause may be a fracture of the wrist, ankle, or hip. Try to remember if your patient has suffered a recent fall. Hip fractures are common in Alzheimer patients in the later stages of dementia. Balance diminishes and gait becomes unsteady, both of which increase the likelihood of a fall.

- Another cause of pain may be ill-fitting dentures. Check your patient for inflamed, red gums. Consult your dentist if you find any mouth problems.

- Anything that causes pain such as headaches, tooth pain, etc. can cause your patient to become angry.

*How can I learn to deal more effectively with my patient's anger or aggression?*

- Don't take anger or aggression personally - your patient is not necessarily angry with you. He or she may be angry for other reasons. You just happen to be there to bear the brunt of the anger.

- Remain calm when your patient is angry. Try searching for the origin of the anger since your patient may not be able to communicate the reason to you.

- Don't ask your patient to "try harder." Alzheimer patients have limited thinking ability, and they can only work within their limitations. Asking them to try harder may actually cause more anger and frustration to surface. Statements such as, "I know you're not angry with me. It's the situation. Let's do something to make the situation better," may help.

- Don't try to win an argument. Instead, try to redirect your patient's thinking processes. For example, if your patient continues to insist that he or she is in Cleveland, but you know that you are both in Florida, there is no harm in allowing your patient to continue thinking that you are in Cleveland. You can redirect the patient's attention from the issue by asking a question such as, "What's the weather like in Cleveland this time of year?"

- Address your patient by his or her first name as often as possible. This has a calming effect that facilitates communication and preserves the patient's dignity.

- Remember that you cannot stop all of your patient's anger, fear, and aggression. Cope as well as you can. Keep in mind that emotional outbursts are disease-related.

*How can I curb angry or aggressive behavior?*

- If anger and aggression occur often, try keeping a daily journal of episodes. Note specifically what precedes the episode. A pattern may emerge that will help you find the cause of the aggressive or angry behavior.

- If undressing for a bath induces aggression in your patient, back away for a few minutes. Try letting your patient perform one small step at a time. For example, you may want to start with, "We'll loosen your shoes so you'll be more comfortable." If your patient still resists undressing, then move on to tooth brushing. Then later, you can suggest undressing for a bath once again.

- If your patient becomes aggressive while performing personal hygiene such as mouth care, divert the anger by asking your patient to hold the toothbrush or tube of toothpaste. Then resume the personal care after a few moments. Your patient may forget why he or she was angry.

- If possible, perform routine care early in the day when Alzheimer patients are less likely to be fatigued.

- If your patient reacts to a situation with anger and you can't seem to divert his or her attention or find the cause of the anger, try the following: clap your hands loudly, then say, "Look! Behind you!" Many patients will quickly forget their anger. If your patient questions you about what was there, you can say that you thought you saw something fall down but must have been mistaken.

- You can sometimes control anger or anxiety by simply giving your patient a favorite doll, teddy bear, or stuffed animal. Also, a soft, cuddly live pet often has a wonderful calming effect on the patient.

- Gently touch your patient. Many Alzheimer patients respond warmly to touch.

### *What activities may help my patient feel less anger and anxiety?*

- Looking through a family photo album may stimulate old, pleasant memories that will have a calming effect on your patient.

- Help your patient keep a personal diary or journal. This promotes routine, preserves memory and lowers overall stress levels in many patients.

- Create a "busy box." Place all kinds of gadgets such as keys, small toy cars, dolls, puzzles, knobs, and things with dials inside the busy box. When your patient becomes angry or anxious, place the busy box nearby.

- Watch a videotape of family members if one is available. These videotapes should be of pleasant events from the past. If you have old 8mm home movies of your family, consider having them transferred to videotape.

- Watch funny commercially made videos that may make your patient laugh such as old Lucille Ball shows, etc. Many local libraries have extensive video collections that can be borrowed free of charge. Make sure these videos don't contain anything that may agitate your patient such as loudness or too much physicality. Watching people on the television may confuse and disturb some patients. They may think that the people on the TV are in the room. Ideally, you should try to watch the TV along with the patient for reassurance.

- Involve your patient in a routine exercise program. Offer this program at the same time each day, if possible.

- Walking is a great exercise for Alzheimer patients. Walking outdoors in bright sunlight also helps produce vitamin D in the skin of older patients, which helps preserve bone strength. Since most diets of the elderly do not provide all the needed vitamin D requirements, this is an added bonus to taking a walk.

- Listening to music or reading may distract your patient from anger.

### *How can I reduce anger at mealtime?*

Since Alzheimer patients still need the company and comfort of people around them, the following methods should prove effective in controlling mealtime anger.

- With anger prior to dinner, say, "We don't enjoy our meal when there is anger. Perhaps you should wait to join us when you feel better." This may dissipate the anger by mealtime.

- With anger during dinnertime, tell the patient that he or she will be excused from the table. Tell your patient that when the anger is gone, he or she will be welcome to join in with others again.

### *How can I handle my patient if he or she becomes paranoid and is overly suspicious of everything I do?*

- If your patient is exhibiting paranoid behavior, maintain a distance at first. Then take small steps forward, facing the patient. Approaching your patient from behind might be interpreted as an attack.
  *Note: A patient who is paranoid and highly suspicious must be handled very carefully.*

- Don't whisper. It may confirm their worst fears.

- Don't mix medications with food in your patient's presence when he or she is in a paranoid state. The patient may interpret this as an attempt to poison them.

- If an item is missing, avoid confrontation about it. Simply offer to help the patient look for it. If your patient is looking for something you know won't be found, look anyway and try distraction to calm the patient.

- White clothing tends to startle Alzheimer patients. Avoid wearing white clothing, if possible.

- Soft music or nature sounds can be useful in calming your patient.

- "White noise" can calm an agitated person. It is a low intensity, repetitive sound such as the whirl of a fan or gentle hum of an air conditioner.

### *Are there any drugs or medications I can use to calm my patient?*

If anger, anxiety, and aggressive behavior become unmanageable, discuss this situation with your patient's physician. Your doctor can make the best choice based on his or her knowledge of your patient and your caregiving situation.

- Your physician may feel that prescription medications are necessary, although they are generally used as a last resort. Haloperidol is commonly prescribed for these types of behavior problems.

- Risperidone is a newer anti-psychotic drug that seems to have fewer side effects than haloperidol.

- Propanolol, carbamazepine and sodium valproate also have been used successfully as an alternative to standard drugs.

- Estrogen in skin patch form has also been used successfully to reduce aggression in about 50% of male Alzheimer patients.

- Benzodiazepines, such as Valium, are generally not used. These drugs tend to increase confusion and the chances of a fall.

- Scopolamine is also known to cause confusion in Alzheimer patients.

# Wandering and the "Safe Return" Program

Wandering is common among Alzheimer patients. It is estimated that more than 50% of Alzheimer patients tend to wander. Although agitation is often associated with wandering, non-agitated patients may also wander. As dementia becomes more severe, wandering tends to increase.

Wandering away from home can result in serious consequences. The National Alzheimer's Association offers a program called *Safe Return* to caregivers and extended care facilities. You only need to register once to remain a member for the life of your patient. This U.S. government-funded program is offered for a one-time fee of $40. A discussion of the *Safe Return* program follows this section.

*Why do some patients wander? What can I do to help to avoid this problem?*

- Boredom is often the cause. Finding interesting activities to fill your patient's time may stop his or her wandering.

- Your patient may be searching for familiar objects. For an Alzheimer patient, familiarity is comforting. Familiar objects such as favorite pieces of furniture, clothing, and pictures should adorn their living area.

- Extroverts wander because they have been social all their lives and continue to enjoy going places and meeting other people. These patients continue to live lifelong habits. Try to involve them with group activities that can fill their need to socialize such as those offered at adult day care centers.

- Stress causes some patients to wander. Look for the triggers in your patient's environment that create stress. See if you can avoid those triggers. Possible stressors might include a change in routine, excessive noise, or exposure to unfamiliar people.

- Fear may cause your patient to leave the immediate area. Your patient may misinterpret a sound or sight. He or she may be trying to get away from it as a way to seek security and safety. If you believe that your patient is hallucinating (seeing or hearing things that are not there) make every effort to keep the patient in the sight of someone in your household at all times.

- Patients may wander if they need to go to the bathroom but do not know or remember where it is. You can help by setting up a regular bathroom schedule that works best for your patient, such as every two hours. Clearly mark the bathroom with a large sign and a picture of a toilet.

*What are some of the dangers of patient wandering?*

You can make your best effort to safeguard your own home for your patient, but if he or she wanders into the neighborhood, there are endless dangers. Swimming pools, yards cluttered with toys and lawn equipment, or unlocked garages with tools and poisonous liquids are a few. Alert your neighbors to a potential wanderer. Ask them to call you immediately if they see your patient outside of the boundaries of your home. Other dangers include:

- Getting lost. Attach ID tags to your patient's clothing and include identification and your address and phone number in your patient's wallet.

- Bumping into objects. Patients increase their chances of injury and falls if they bump into objects because they are in an unfamiliar surrounding.

*What are some preventative measures I can take if my patient is a wanderer?*

Doors and doorknobs can be a safety problem. Your patient may not realize that a door is an exit. Here are several solutions.

- To hide a doorknob, cover the doorknob with cloth close in color to the door. Secure the cloth to the door with Velcro.

- Hang a picture over a doorknob to disguise it.

- Using black tape, place a series of black horizontal grids on the floor in front of the door. This pattern discourages Alzheimer patients from coming near it.

- At home or especially in crowded places, have your patient wear a belt (even if the garment doesn't require one). A belt will allow you to quickly grab your patient if he or she is about to exit a door.

- Install motion detectors near doors and have them wired to set off an alarm.

- Purchase or rent a wander alarm. You'll find suppliers listed in Appendix C.

*What safety measures can I take to protect my wandering patient?*

- Obtain a medical bracelet from your local jeweler or drug store. Have the ID bracelet engraved to read, "I AM AN ALZHEIMER PATIENT." Provide the caregiver's address and telephone number. (Keep area code changes up-to-date.)

- Alert your neighbors and police department that you have an Alzheimer patient at home. If they see your patient away from your home unaccompanied, they will know immediate action is necessary. Give the neighbors your telephone number, *especially* if it is unlisted.

- Make a video of your Alzheimer patient so the police will have a helpful tool to locate your patient if he or she becomes lost or missing. Keep a good current picture available. Have photocopies ready to pass around in the area.

- Keep an *unwashed* item of clothing that belongs to your patient on hand. Police dogs may be able to locate your loved one from the scent left on the clothing.

- Sew bicycle reflectors or highly reflective fabric on clothing that your patient wears outdoors. If the patient wanders off at night, he or she will be more visible to drivers. These products often can be found in sporting good stores, bicycle shops, or craft and fabric stores.

- Identification information can be written on iron-on clothing labels.

### How can I channel my patient's need to wander into something positive?

- Go for walks with your patient. Let your patient lead the way whenever possible. Walking is good exercise for Alzheimer patients. Walking increases appetite, increases blood circulation, and also helps prevent contractures, which are the painful shortening of muscles.

- If you have a patient who loves to wander and is not agitated by crowds, take them to a shopping mall and walk with him or her.
  *Note: Know where the mall exits, elevators, and escalators are located.*

- If your patient is not comfortable in crowds, call your local shopping mall to ask about their pre-opening hours walking program. Many malls now open early to allow senior citizens to freely exercise before mall-shopping crowds arrive.

- When you are out walking, have your patient wear a slightly loose-fitting belt. A grip on the belt will give you better control than holding your patient's hand or arm.

### What is the Alzheimer Association's Safe Return program?

*Safe Return* is the only nationwide identity program for Alzheimer patients. The program operates through the National Alzheimer's Association. Since 1993, more than 72,000 patients have been registered. More than 97% of registered patients who have wandered away have been located and returned to their families. Joining *Safe Return* before your patient begins to wander is a sound idea.

### How does the Safe Return program work?

- Once you register with the program, you supply the National Alzheimer's Association with a photograph of your patient and it becomes part of a national photo information database.

- You will receive wandering behavior education and training along with the telephone number of a 24-hour toll-free emergency crisis line.

- You will be supplied with your choice of an ID bracelet or necklace, iron-on clothing labels, wallet ID, key chain ID, and lapel pins for your patient to wear.

- Once a patient is reported missing by a caregiver or family member, *Safe Return* immediately alerts local law enforcement agencies. Photo flyers can be created and faxed to law enforcement personnel and hospitals to aid in the search.

- Local Alzheimer's Association chapters provide families with support while searches are conducted.

### *How do I register for the program?*

There are several ways to register or learn more about the program. Choose the one that is most convenient for you.

- Register for *Safe Return* by calling the National Alzheimer's Association at 1-800-272-3900. You will be asked to fill out a simple form.

- Visit the National Alzheimer Association's website at **www.alz.org**. A list of local chapters is available at that site under "Programs and Resources." You may register through your local chapter.

- Call *Safe Return* directly at the toll-free number 1-888-572-8566.

- Many family physicians have information on registration for *Safe Return*.

### *Do care facilities participate in the Safe Return Program?*

- Many care facilities already have their Alzheimer patients registered in *Safe Return*. Check to make sure the one you use has this service.

- Many adult day care centers require Alzheimer patients using their facilities to already be part of *Safe Return*.

### *How much does it cost to join Safe Return?*

As of the year 2001, there is a one-time-only fee of $40. That fee entitles your patient to a lifetime membership.

*Chapter Topics and Suggested Readings*
*from the Alzheimer's Association 2001 Public Publications Catalog:*

*Communicating*

Communicating – VHS video

Steps to Enhancing Communications: Interacting with Persons with Alzheimer's
Disease – brochure

Steps for Caregivers: Caring for Persons with Alzheimer's Disease – audiotape –
Includes: Steps to Enhancing Communications, Steps to Understanding
Challenging Behaviors – narrated by Shelly Fabares

*Managing Anger and Aggression*

Combativeness – fact sheet

Hallucinations – fact sheet

Managing Difficult Behavior – VHS video

Steps to Understanding Challenging Behavior - brochure

*Wandering and the Safe Return Program*

Wandering – fact sheet

Steps to Ensuring Safety: Preventing Wandering and Getting Lost – brochure

Safe Return – brochure

# Chapter Four


## Guarding Against Bodily Harm
## ~
## Safety Issues


~ *" A good head and a good heart are always
a formidable combination"* ~

Nelson Mandela

# Preventing At-Home Injuries

An Alzheimer patient needs protection from danger in much the same way a child needs protection. As memory impairment progresses, your patient will require heavy supervision. With the unpredictable nature of dementia, continuous scrutiny of your home will be necessary to keep your patient out of harm's way.

It can be a difficult task to anticipate new dangers lurking in every room of your home. A home safety check is essential. If many years have passed since you've done such a check, the following information can help you safeguard your patient.

Accidents happen even in the safest homes. Keeping a good first aid kit available will prepare you for the unexpected. Make sure the kit is handy and that medications and ointments, etc. are not outdated.

A simple, but often overlooked, safety precaution is to make sure that emergency telephone numbers are available at a moment's notice. Contact numbers for your patient's physician, the poison control center, local police number other than 911 should be within your reach. Keep a list of people who can stay with your patient if an emergency arises that means you have to leave. Keep a list of those who could drive you and your patient somewhere if necessary. Make sure all these contact numbers are current.

## How can I make my home safer?

- All windows in your home should be secured and locked, especially as dementia increases. Many hardware stores sell simple window clamps that prevent a window from opening up far enough to allow someone to fall out.

- Keep extension cords away from areas where your patient walks. Remember that an Alzheimer patient's visual perception is impaired.

- Keep clotheslines high enough that your patient will not walk into them. He or she could possibly choke on a clothesline. If possible, take down clotheslines when not in use.

- Low-hanging plants can be a hazard. Hang plants high above areas where your patient may be walking.

- Remove the lock from the bathroom door.

- Install grab bars in shower and tub areas. (See Appendix D)

- Use low-intensity showerheads with on/off switches (see Appendix D). An intense water flow from a showerhead could startle the patient resulting in a sudden fall.

- Bath mats should have suction cups. Non-slip strips should be placed in the tub and shower.

- Low level glass tabletops are a real hazard to Alzheimer patients. Relocate these away from areas where your patient spends time.

- Keep stairs clutter free. Make sure railings are not loose and can support your patient's weight. Install gates at the top and bottom of stairs.

- Keep bare floors unwaxed. Highly polished floors increase the risk of falls. Also shiny floors may be interpreted as water by your patient. He or she may refuse to walk on it.

- Remove scatter rugs from the home.

### How can I safeguard my patient against hot water burns?

- Always check the temperature of your patient's bath water before you allow the water to touch his or her skin.

- Lower the temperature of your hot water heater. Many Alzheimer patients cannot sense water temperature against their skin very well. Consequently, they could be easily scalded.

- Purchase a device that installs on faucets that helps prevent accidental scalding. (See Appendix D)

- Paint hot water faucet handles red to eliminate confusion.

### What can I do to eliminate safety hazards in the kitchen?

- Don't allow an Alzheimer patient to use the stove.

- Always check the temperature of food before serving it to your patient. Make sure the food is not too hot. With microwaved food, be sure there are no hotspots – stir the food well before serving it.

- Disconnect the garbage disposal. Some patients try to use the disposal as a hiding place for all kinds of items.

- Keep matches out of your patient's reach.

- Unplug appliances such as toasters and electric mixers at nights.

- Keep a loaded fire extinguisher handy to reach in the kitchen. Learn how to use it.

- Lock away potentially poisonous cleaners.

*What other ways can I safeguard my patient at home?*

- Keep all medicines (over-the-counter and prescription) out of your patient's reach. Place them in a specially marked container and keep them hidden away.

- If you have any potentially poisonous houseplants get rid of them. Do some research. Get a list of poisonous plants from your poison control center.

- Store solvents and cleaning fluids away from patients. Your patient may think that a solvent is something to drink. Remember to check the kitchen, bathroom, garage, workshop or anywhere you store such materials. Ideally, these products should be locked up.

- Place child safety plugs on all electrical outlets. Some Alzheimer patients put their fingers or an object such as scissors in the outlet socket holes.

- Consider removing lock tumblers from your patient's room. Otherwise, he or she could accidentally get locked inside.

- Do not allow an Alzheimer patient to smoke, if possible. Never allow your patient to smoke in bed.

- Remove guns from your property to avoid serious gun-related mishaps or injuries. If you don't remove them, lock guns securely away in a cabinet.

*How can I keep my patient safe in the car?*

- Never leave an Alzheimer patient alone in a car. The patient could touch the handbrake and mistakenly release it, or catch their hands in a power window. *Note: Many potentially dangerous accidents could result from a patient being left alone in a vehicle.*

- Always secure your patient's seat belt. The back seat is the safest place for an Alzheimer patient.

- Keep car doors locked.

- Discard car litter such as old cigarettes, coins, pencils, etc.

- Tape down window and door handles or buttons.

# Reducing the Incidence of Injuries from Falling

Falling is common among Alzheimer patients for several reasons. Most falls occur because Alzheimer patients walk more slowly, with shorter strides, and have both impaired vision and depth perception. It is important to do all you can to help your patient avoid falling because that often results in hip fractures.

### What are some medical reasons that make my patient prone to falling?

- Certain medications may increase the risk of falling such as sleeping pills, sedatives, or benzodiazepines. Check with your pharmacist, nurse, or the patient's physician about possible side effects from medications.

- Transient strokes also occur in Alzheimer patients. This type of stroke can cause a patient to fall frequently. Contact your physician immediately if the patient shows signs of stumbling or falling repeatedly for no apparent reason.

### Is there anything I can do to help my patient avoid a fall or to soften the blow from a fall?

- When walking with your patient, try grasping his or her belt from behind or curl up the back of the patient's shirt and grasp it to help prevent a fall.

- Some home health stores carry hip pads that can be worn by the patient to help prevent hip fractures if a fall occurs. Hip pads can greatly decrease the incidence of fractures.

- For your patient's eyeglasses, choose plastic lenses instead of glass, if possible. Broken glass lenses could possibly injure the patient if he or she falls.

### Are there some visual clues I can give my patient to help prevent a fall?

- Place brightly colored tape on the edge of stair steps. This will draw the patient's attention to the edges of the stairs.

- Paint hot water faucets red to help the patient distinguish between hot and cold spigots.

- Use visual contrasts whenever possible. For example, use dark-colored door-knobs on light-colored doors. (Remember – these door knobs may need camouflaging if wandering is a problem.)

- Remove mirrors from the backs of doors. Some patients interpret a mirror as an empty space and may try to walk through it.

*What types of products can I use in my home to help avoid falls?*

- Use non-skid mats on any tile surfaces. Don't use high luster polish on these surfaces.

- Nightlights inserted into electrical sockets should be used to keep hallways well lighted.

- Use plastic-molded furniture with rounded edges in the areas where your patient spends a good deal of time.  If a fall occurs, they may help minimize injuries.

## Taking Away the Car Keys
## Should Your Patient Be Driving?

Telling an Alzheimer patient that he or she should not drive a vehicle often meets with a great deal of resistance and anger. But most Alzheimer patients should not be driving. Driving becomes hazardous when a patient's dementia causes changes in visual perception and impaired judgment. The following statistics reveal the dangers involved in allowing an Alzheimer patient to continue to drive.

- In a recent study, a test was designed using 20 different kinds of traffic signs. Elderly subjects who were free of the disease correctly recognized 15 of the 20 signs. Conversely, mildly demented Alzheimer patients correctly recognized only 8 of the 20 signs.

- The Alzheimer's Association, warns "individuals with dementia are twice as likely to be involved in a traffic accident as other persons the same age."

- More than 50% of all Alzheimer patients stop driving within 3 years of their diagnosis.

(A Personal Note from Author Jim Knittweis) "When my father had Alzheimer's, he resented anyone telling him that he should not drive. I handled the issue in a way that gave him a choice. You may want to consider this approach with your loved one. My father was no longer able to read a newspaper or a book at his stage of deterioration when we discussed his driving ability. I obtained a copy of our state's driving manual and told him that he would have to read the manual so that he could pass his upcoming driving test. After my father tried unsuccessfully to read the manual, he decided that he should not drive. By giving him the choice, he voluntarily gave up driving."

*Is there a "test" I can use to let me know if it's time for my patient to stop driving?*

- Draw a stop sign without the word "STOP" written on it. Ask your patient to tell you what the sign means. If he or she can't identify the octagonal shape as a stop sign, then the patient should not be driving.

*What warning signs tell me that it's time to take away the keys?*

According to the Alzheimer's Association, one or more the following behaviors may mean that you have to limit or stop your patient from driving. If your patient:

- Can't locate familiar places

- No longer observes traffic signs

- Is slow to make decisions in traffic

- Makes poor decisions while driving in traffic

- Doesn't quite know what to do at intersections

- Becomes angry or confused while driving

***What can I do if my patient resists giving up driving after I believe he or she should stop?***

Even though it may seem deceptive to use the following tactics, you must consider the lives of your patient, his or her passengers, as well as other motorists and pedestrians. A few options are:

- Ask your physician to give your patient a prescription order to stop driving.

- Sell the car

- Hide the car keys

- Have a "kill" switch installed in the car by an auto mechanic. The car will not start unless the switch is first turned on. Don't tell your patient about the kill switch. He or she will not be able to start the car – even with the keys.

***How can I help make the transition from driving less traumatic for my patient?***

- Reassure your patient that you or someone else will be available when they need a ride.

- Explain other alternatives to your patient such as public transportation or community driving services (check with your local or county Office of Aging).

## Chapter Topics and Suggested Readings
## from the Alzheimer's Association 2001 Public Publications Catalog:

*Preventing At-Home Injuries & Reducing the Incidence of Injury From Falls*

Steps to Enhancing Your Home: Modifying the Environment – brochure
Steps for Caregivers:  Caring for Persons with Alzheimer's Disease – audiotape
  Includes the above discussion among other subjects.
Safety – fact sheet
Safety First – VHS video

*Taking the Car Keys Away – Should Your Patient Be Driving?*

Driving – fact sheet

# Chapter Five

## Maintaining
## Quality Of Life

~ *"In the depth of winter, I finally learned there was in me an invincible summer"* ~

Albert Camus

# Activities To Stimulate Mind and Body

Ideal activities for Alzheimer patients are those that take advantage of old memories and skills, those that require social interaction, and those that promote physical as well as mental activity.

Activities should be broken down into a series of small steps whenever possible. This will allow your patient to more easily understand the activity and will help your patient gain enjoyment from participating in the activity.

### What kinds of activities take advantage of old skills and memories?

- Activities resembling those that a patient once did as a hobby or as a job. For example, if your patient worked as a landscaper or enjoyed gardening, then he or she might enjoy planting seeds or watering individual plants, flowers, or herbs.

- Some patients may have enjoyed making craft projects before their illness. Even though they may no longer be capable of fine motor work, they may still be able to help you hold small parts for gluing.

- If woodworking was a skill enjoyable to your patient, he or she can try sanding wood with various grits of sandpaper.

- Many patients will remember old friends, good times, and dates by looking at old pictures. Help your patient make a photo album. This remembering process is good for your patient's mind. If he or she doesn't remember the people in old pictures, tell stories about those people. For example, you can say, "This is your son, John, when he was 5 years old.  He loved playing baseball with you."

- Construct a memory box. Use a large cardboard box to hold items from your patient's past. An old baseball glove, a favorite book, wedding pictures, an old favorite garment – almost anything with memories attached. Periodically, examine the contents of the box with your patient. Help your patient recall what each item is and what it meant in the past.  Add new items whenever possible to help keep your patient's mind sharp. Allow your patient to collect and add new items to the box.

### Are there any reading-related activities my patient might enjoy?

A note on eyeglasses: Make sure you have more than one pair available for your patient and that you have a copy of your patient's eyeglass prescription on hand. Properly prescribed eyeglasses are not only helpful for reading but are essential to a person with impaired balance, depth perception, and increasing vision problems.

- For patients who still can read, a good idea is the creation of a Worry Book. Alzheimer patients have normal worries and fears. Often, when you explain why patients should not worry about a particular thing, their memory fails them. Ten minutes later, they forget the conversation. They will begin to worry about the same issue all over again. Entering each worry in the Worry Book may avoid this problem for your patient. Next to each worry, write the reason why this worry is not valid. For example, if your patient is worried about money, write on the money page how all the money is being prudently taken care of. Then each time the money worry surfaces, your patient can simply read the Worry Book for comfort. The Worry Book is a great frustration saver.

- Some patients can be kept busy looking at newspapers or magazines for coupons. If possible, let your patient sort the coupons. It will help if you first stack a few sample coupons on the table so your patient can glance over and remember what he or she is looking for.

- Help your patient cut pictures from favorite magazines. You may want to tie your choice of pictures to an old hobby that the patient enjoyed such as floral arranging. Have your patient cut out pictures of flowers and then paste them in a scrapbook.

- Read stories together. It's a great way to share special moments. (Some Alzheimer patients have problems with vision. Often, they cannot verbalize their inability to read. This activity is a good way to watch for the need of a vision check.)

- Another good activity to stimulate memory is to write a word on an index card and then let the patient glue a picture of the word on the back. Use words that are related to food, clothing, and other daily activities. For example, one card may feature a picture of a key. Show the word "key" to the patient and ask your patient to tell you what it means. If he or she has trouble identifying the word, turn the back of the card around and show your patient the picture of the key. Often the picture will help the patient to recall the word. Keep the card collection in a 3" x 5" file card box.

- Ask your patient to sort playing cards by suit or number.

### What activities will help promote outdoor physical exercise and mental stimulation for my patient?

- As mentioned previously, walking is an excellent exercise. A regular walking program improves sleep at night, improves mood, increases communication, and decreases agitation. You also can stimulate your patient's mind by helping him or her notice and remember the names of common sights such as a neighbor's home or a traffic light during your walk.

- In the spring season, stroll through the yard with your patient. Let your patient help you decide where to plant your garden or flowers.

- Allow your patient to help with gardening chores such as weeding or picking fruits and vegetables from the vines. Regardless of the size of your garden, your patient can take great joy in being part of the process.

- Encourage your patient to help rake leaves in the autumn. Discuss the different colors of the falling leaves.

### What are some activities that will help promote fine motor skills for my patient?

- Sorting coins and placing them in the appropriate wrappers.

- Sorting buttons by color and size, then placing them in separate containers.

- Removing shells from peanuts.

- Polishing silverware. This routine occupies a great deal of time.

- Stringing various sized and colored beads together.

### Should I encourage my patient to participate in daily chores?

Yes. Routine, repetitive activity is ideal for Alzheimer patients. Some suggestions are:

- Sorting and folding clothing.

- Stacking dirty dishes in the sink.

- Helping to make cookies – the patient can stir the dough.

- Helping to shine shoes.

- Caring for a pet, if you have one. The care of your pet should be the patient's responsibility to whatever extent he or she can handle these duties.

# Travel Suggestions and Precautions

Traveling with an Alzheimer patient can be very frustrating both to the patient and to the caregiver as well. There are times when the caregiver badly needs a vacation. Many fine elder day care or respite care centers are available where a patient can be well cared for while the caregiver gets a much-needed rest. But if you are taking your patient on vacation, here are a few ideas to help make a trip as comfortable as possible for all.

*How can I help our travel experience to be as comfortable as possible?*

- Spend as little time as possible on noisy planes, in crowded airport terminals, and near people speaking foreign languages. All these tend to annoy Alzheimer patients.

- When flying, try to avoid connecting flights. This process is disruptive to many Alzheimer patients.

- Consider taking your patient on vacation in a rented motor home. Unfamiliar accommodations can make patients agitated. A motor home is ideal since it will offer a similar environment for the patient each night.

- Bring plenty of extra underwear and incontinence pads.

- Bring some familiar things along for the patient such as a favorite magazine, puzzle, or knitting project.

- Bring several nightlights along when traveling. Use them at your lodging accommodations.

- Taking a companion along on a trip is a good idea. Your companion can keep an eye on the luggage while you help your patient in the restroom facilities.

*What should I do if my patient is of the opposite sex and we need to use public bathroom facilities?*

- When traveling, look for a one-person type restroom for your patient. It is easier, less stressful, and more private for your patient. However, these types of restrooms are not always available.

- The U. S. Government's Americans with Disabilities Act (ADA) policy in regard to using public restrooms if you are of the opposite sex of your patient is: a public place such as a restaurant, rest area, airport, convention center, etc., should use "reasonable modification to policy, practices, and procedures." Simply put, it means that you should ask the management to allow you, the caretaker, to accompany your patient into the restroom used by your gender.

The facility manager should make every reasonable accommodation for you. Many airports and other large public places have unisex bathrooms. But, if you can't find one, ask to speak to the manager of that building. Call the ADA information line at 1-800-514-0301 for any policy information.

### When traveling, whom should I notify of our special status?

- Tell your tour guide that your companion has Alzheimer disease.

- When visiting museums, tourist attractions, etc., carry a card that states, "My companion has Alzheimer disease. Please direct all questions to me."

- Travel officials and tour guides should be notified of other special needs. For example, is your patient hearing- or vision-impaired? Is your patient prone to falls? These are the types of concerns to which you should alert officials.

- If you are staying at a motel, let management know you have an Alzheimer patient staying with you who may wander from the premises. Then staff members will know to immediately notify you if they see your patient alone.

- If you think your patient may become disruptive on public transportation, notify the driver or crew members beforehand. Assure them that you will do all you can to keep disruptions to a minimum.

### Are there any special precautions I should remember?

- Never send an Alzheimer patient on a trip alone on a plane, train, or bus.

- If you stay overnight in a motel, consider taking a portable door alarm with you. The alarm will trigger when the door is open. Then you will be alerted if your patient should wander. These devices can be purchased in electronic stores.

- Carry a current picture of your patient with you in case your patient wanders or becomes separated from you at any time.

- Make sure your patient is wearing identification information.

- Include the *Safe Return* telephone number on your patient's identification information (if you have registered for the program).

# Avoiding Fatigue in the Alzheimer Patient

Alzheimer patients fatigue easily. Morning and early afternoon may be their best times for activities. By late evening, many patients become irritable, frustrated and have numerous behavior problems. This behavior change in late evening is known as "sundowning."

### How can I manage patient fatigue?

- Alzheimer patients should sit quietly in a recliner for about 40 minutes at 10 a.m., then for about 90 minutes at 2 p.m. You can use quilts or blankets as a cue to mark rest periods. Don't have visitors and don't offer coffee to your patient before or during these times.

- Give your patient frequent breaks in activity with as many naps as necessary.

- Instead of one long activity, break up the day into a series of small activities.

- Plan short trips. All-day travel to a distant place or relative's home may be especially fatiguing to your patient.

## Chapter Topics and Suggested Readings
### from the Alzheimer's Association 2001 Public Publications Catalog:

*Activities to Stimulate Mind and Body*

Steps to Planning Activities: Structuring the Day at Home – brochure
Steps for Caregivers: Caring for Persons with Alzheimer's Disease – audiotape
      Includes the above subject as well as other topics
Activities – fact sheet

*Travel Suggestions and Precautions*

Vacationing – fact sheet
Visiting – fact sheet

# Chapter Six

## The Common Bonds
## of Caregiving

*~ "Experience is not what happens to you;
it's what you do with what happens to you" ~*

Aldous Huxley

# Family Issues

Alzheimer caregiving brings great changes to family dynamics. Each family learns to cope with a loved one with this disease in its own unique way, as does each individual within the family. But many caregivers face similar problems, ask similar questions, and share many of the same concerns.

Based on extensive research, we know what problems caregivers wrestle with most often and we offer solutions to these problems.

*Is there a lack of information available to Alzheimer caregivers?*

- Yes. Many families believe the information that they receive from medical doctors and other health professionals leaves them unprepared to cope with the behavioral consequences of Alzheimer's.

*Where can I find information?*

- We are in the midst of an information explosion. The Internet is an endless source of information about Alzheimer's. If you do not have a computer or are reluctant to use one, ask a friend or family member to do some computer search for you. (See Appendix B - *Resources For Caregivers*, which includes advice on how to evaluate the validity of health-related websites.)

- The Alzheimer's Association is ready and able to help caregivers in a myriad of ways. Many of their pamphlets and informational materials are offered in English and in Spanish. You can visit their website (www.alz.org) or call their national headquarters at 800-272-3900 for information or to find a local chapter near you.

*What is the most common problem facing caregivers?*

The problem most often mentioned is the patient's need for constant supervision. The inability to leave home to shop or do chores causes caregivers tremendous mental strain.

*How can a caregiver get relief from this problem?*

- Don't be shy about asking other family members to relieve you, if only for a few hours. Plan an activity for your patient and the temporary caregiver such as taking a walk or sharing a meal. The more specific the request, the easier it will be to fulfill.

- Check into adult day care facilities for your patient. Don't be too quick to think that your patient won't do well at a day care facility. Many Alzheimer patients actually enjoy the company of other patients.

*What other daily problems do caregivers face?*

- Patient wandering

- The many tasks involved in the patient's activities of daily living

*Where can I find help for these problems?*

- Join the Alzheimer Association's *Safe Return* program. (See Chapter 3 for details)

- Many local Alzheimer's Association chapters offer a free 8-hour intensive family caregiver training session at least once a year. Learning how to cope with your patient's activities of daily living can lighten caregiver burden.

*What family-related issues will I face?*

More than half of all caregivers say that conflict within their family is a major source of stress. Many of these conflicts are brought on by differences of opinion concerning:

- How to care for the patient.

- Family member actions or attitudes toward the patient.

- Attitudes or actions by one family member to another. Often, one member will complain that other members are not shouldering their share of the care.

- The stages of grief and perception of loss felt by individual family members. These experiences can be different in length and severity for individuals.

- The need for nursing home placement for the patient.

*How can I find a way to avoid or resolve these conflicts?*

- Family counseling is very helpful. A great deal of good can result from a group airing of problems with an objective mediator leading the discussion.

- Remind yourself and other family members that individual responses to the grief process and how each person becomes reconciled to the disease can cause misinterpretation of attitude among those members.

- Join the National Family Caregivers Association (NFCA). The association was created to support, educate, and empower Americans caring for chronically ill loved ones. Membership is free to family caregivers. It can be reached at **www.nfcacares.org** or call 800-896-3650. The address is 10400 Connecticut Ave., #500, Kensington, MD 20895. Many free pamphlets and guidebooks are available to members.

- Openly discuss the possibility that your loved one may need nursing home placement. Start this discussion among family members when your patient is diagnosed with Alzheimer's. Make the decision for nursing home placement a family decision. Learn all you can about nursing homes in your area (see Appendix C – *Choosing a Nursing Home*).

# Financial Issues

A person with Alzheimer's may forget, become confused, or be very secretive about his or her assets. You will have to identify these assets to determine how much money is available for caregiving needs. Many financial and legal issues regarding your patient's sources of income and your ability to draw on these funds for patient care will arise.

Money always is a touchy family issue. But the primary caregiver needs access to the patient's bank accounts, etc. to help safeguard the patient's assets and to meet the patient's healthcare needs over an undetermined amount of time.

## Where can I look to find information about my patient's financial assets

Gather as much asset information as possible. Items to look for include:
- Bank statements, savings pass books, canceled checks
- Insurance policies
- Wills and trusts
- Credit cards and past statements
- Safe deposit box keys

Check for possible income from the following sources:
- Any salaries owed to the patient from an employer
- Pension (employer or military) or Social Security income
- Stocks, mutual funds, bonds, or annuities
- Disability benefits from insurance policies
- Real estate or valuable personal property such as jewelry or antiques

## What kind of healthcare-related financial burdens will I encounter?

- Funding for adult day care
- Home health care
- Respite programs
- Nursing home funds
- Long-term health care insurance

*How can I meet the high cost of caring for my patient?*

- Check with Medicaid, Medicare, the Social Security Administration. Contact the U.S. Department of Health & Human Services for Medicaid and Medicare information at **www.os.dhhs.gov** or call 877-696-6775 (toll free). Contact the Social Security Administration at **www.ssa.gov** or call 800-772-1213.

- If your patient is a U.S. military veteran, contact the Department of Veterans Affairs. He or she may qualify for medical care and prescription drug benefits. For eligibility, call the VA Health Benefits Service Center at 877-222-8387 (toll free) or visit their website at **www.va.gov.**

- Go through your patient's records of insurance. He or she may have coverage for long-term health care. Call insurance companies, ask for information.

- If your patient is elderly, check with the Internal Revenue Service (IRS) about possible tax benefits. Ask for any tax booklets relating to older Americans.

*Where can I turn for financial help with my patient's medication costs?*

Expenses for patient medications such as new Alzheimer drugs or routine prescription medicines not covered by insurance can be expensive or even beyond the range of your patient's income and assets. Check with the following:

- The Pharmaceutical Research and Manufacturers of America at **www.phrma.org** or call 202-835-3400 to see if your patient qualifies for their free prescription drugs program.

- Your local or county social services office to see if any financial assistance is available for the cost of medications.

*What sources do I have for help with the legalities of financial issues?*

- Check with the National Senior Citizens Law Center at **www.nsclc.org** or call 202-289-6976. This nonprofit group advocates for legal rights for older individuals with disabilities and for low-income elderly.

- The National Academy of Elder Law Attorneys offers publications on elder law recourses and questions you should ask when choosing an attorney. Contact them at **www.naela.com** or call 520-881-4005. An attorney will be valuable to help you prepare living wills, durable powers of attorney, and estate planning for your patient.

- The AARP also offers valuable information about legal issues, home health care, and nursing home issues. Contact them at **www.aarp.org** or call 800-424-3410.

*What are some of the financial and legal terms I should know and understand?*

Just as in other areas of patient care, your patient's financial and legal needs will change as the disease process progresses. In our Glossary, which was taken from the Alzheimer's Association Glossary, you will find a list of financial and legal terms. They are important for you to know and understand. Here is additional information you should know to safeguard your patient's finances:

- Joint bank accounts – at some point, you may need the type of accounts that can be used for deposit or withdrawal of funds by either co-owner. It is essential that it be stated that owner A *or* owner B can make transactions on the account. This type of account is important for money management by the primary caregiver and is often already in place with spouses. But if someone other than a spouse is the primary caregiver, make sure that caregiver has access to the patient's funds for bill paying, etc.

- Wills for spouses – both spouses should have a will that has been signed and reviewed by an attorney. If the spouse of the patient were to die first, it should be assured that funds would be left in trust for the benefit and care of the surviving spouse who is ill. *Always consult an attorney about legal issues.*

- Testamentary capacity – refers to the legal competence to know one is making a will, including what property is to be distributed and the names and relationships of those named to be beneficiaries of the property.

*Chapter Topics and Suggested Readings*
*from the Alzheimer's Association 2001 Public Publications Catalog:*

### Family Issues

Alone but Not Forgotten: A Providers' Manual – also in VHS video
      (for caregivers of patients living alone)
Caring for the Caregiver - Especially for the Alzheimer Caregiver
      — VHS 20-minute video
Especially for the Alzheimer Caregiver – brochure
Helping Children and Teens Understand Alzheimer's Disease – brochure
How to Be a Long-Distance Caregiver – brochure
Living with Early-Onset Alzheimer's Disease
      (family relationships and finances) - brochure
Steps for Caregivers: Caring for Persons with Alzheimer's Disease – audiotape
Telling the Patient, Family, and Friends – fact sheet

### Financial Issues

Services You May Need (medical, financial, and care services) - brochure
Steps to Understanding Financial Issues: Resources for Caregivers - brochure
Steps to Understanding Legal Issues: Planning for the Future - brochure
Taxes and Alzheimer's Disease - brochure
Understanding Medicaid Long-Term Care - guide
Private Long-Term Insurance Care - guide
Know Your Rights to Cure and Treatment in a Nursing Home - guide

# Chapter Seven

## Caregiver Stress

~ "To endure is greater than to dare; to tire out
of hostile fortune; to be daunted
by no difficulty; to keep heart when
all have lost it - who can say
this is not greatness?" ~

William Makepeace Thackeray

*How Caregiver Stress is Measured*
*What Causes It*
*How To Cope With It*

The stress of Alzheimer caregiving has many roots. A profound sadness for the loss of normalcy in your life as well as in the life of your loved one is its foundation. As time passes, a sense of isolation from your social circle begins to take a toll. And the daily frustrations of watching a loved one spiral downward into a process of unlearning wears away a caregiver's spirit.

But the human spirit is resilient. We rise to the occasion time and again. We call upon our inner strength to find ways to solve problems and renew ourselves. Gaining back our innate fortitude can happen. It happens through the awareness of a withering spirit. As a caregiver, you can empower yourself by accepting that stress is an undeniable companion but one that can be controlled.

Researchers use the term "caregiver burden" to describe caregiver stress. By not allowing caregiver burden to gather enough strength to leave you vulnerable, you can lessen the likelihood of health problems or depression.

*How burdened do caregivers feel?*

Studies have shown that caregiver burden is a problem for the vast majority of Alzheimer caregivers. The extent of the burden depends on how much and what kind of support the caregiver receives.

*How can I tell how much caregiver burden I am experiencing?*

Various tests have been designed to measure caregiver burden. We suggest that you take the Zarit Burden Interview. This test was designed by Steven Zarit, Ph.D., author of many Alzheimer-related books. It is simple to use and score.

*Where can I find the Zarit Burden Interview?*

- At the end of this chapter.

- The test can be obtained by e-mail at no charge. Requests go to **syh1@psu.edu.**

*What factors contribute to the degree of burden felt by caregivers?*

- Caregivers living with their patient have the highest burden scores.

- Angry, resentful caregivers consistently report feeling more burdened than those not reporting these feelings.

- Caregivers in ill health report higher perceived burden.

*What can I do to relieve the burden caused by these problems?*

- Learn to delegate the responsibilities of household chores to other family members. Since the primary caregiver carries the most burden, he or she must find a way to lighten the load. Ask family members to:

  - Prepare meals that can be frozen for later use.

  - Set aside a few hours each week to help you with chores such as laundry, even if it means taking the laundry to their house and returning it to you.

  - Run errands such as trips to the drug store or supermarket. It is far simpler for another family member to go to the store without having to take the patient along each time.

- Gain control of your feelings of anger and resentment by acknowledging them. Women are good at expressing their feelings. But they are not as willing to own up to negative feelings. Both women and men will gain control of these emotions by openly discussing them with professional counselors, family members, friends, or support group members.

*What are some of the causes of caregiver burden in women?*

- Although women air their feelings more often than men, they tend to avoid confrontation and readily accept personal blame for problems that arise from caregiving.

- Women approach tasks by using "enfolding." They combine tasks and try to do too many things at once. This approach can lead to the feeling that you never completely accomplish anything.

- Numerous studies show women care for more severely demented patients than do male caregivers. Caregiver burden increases as dementia worsens.

*What can women do to relieve caregiver burden?*

- Be honest with yourself – you are not Superwoman. Recognize that you are only one person and can only do so much.

- Stop blaming yourself for everything negative that happens with your patient. Women should remember that many caregiving problems are inherent in the situation and beyond their control.

- Learn to be more assertive. Asking for a helping hand before problems become overwhelming is the part of a situation that can be controlled.

- Make the choice of nursing home placement a family decision. The burden of caring for a severely demented patient often occurs because women are so reluctant to place a loved one in a nursing home. A sense of responsibility and guilt play into this difficult decision. To make that choice a family decision can relieve guilt and caregiver burden in the later stages of the disease process.

*What are some of the causes of caregiver burden in men?*

- Most male caregivers say they feel socially isolated and are deeply affected by the loss of female companionship.

- Men express a need to talk to other men. Subjects they would like to discuss include issues involving sexual relations, platonic female friendships, and the personal hygiene of their wives.

- Men often view asking for help as a sign of weakness. Male caregivers tend to try caring for their wives without help from others. Most make no demands on or have expectations of help from their children.

- Men approach caregiving in a "take charge" manner. Generally, men are more proficient in tasks such as money management and household repairs than in the more traditional female roles of carrying out personal care activities such as dressing, bathing, and grooming their patient.

*What can men do about these problems?*

- Attend a support group where you feel comfortable openly discussing sensitive issues such as sexual intimacy. These groups can also provide the much-needed companionship that men lack when their wives become ill.

- Delegate those chores that you are not comfortable with to female family members, housekeepers, or home health aides. Or, ask a female family member or friend for advice on how to handle these aspects of caregiving.

*How does the caregiver's attitude toward the patient contribute to perceived burden?*

- Caregivers who attribute their patient's behavior to the patient's illness are less burdened than caregivers who attribute the patient's behavior to patient willfulness.

- Those who see the patient as "emotionally demanding" or "dependent" feel a higher sense of burden than those who see the patient as "disturbed" or "disabled."

- Caring for a very forgetful patient is perceived as a higher burden than caring for a patient with mild forgetfulness.

*How can I change my attitude if it is creating caregiver burden?*

- Change your perception through education. How caregivers perceive a stressor helps to modify the amount of burden felt. Learn about the disease process and how it affects caregiving through reading, viewing videos, and going to support groups. It is a fact that caregivers have a limited amount of time. But taking time to learn how to deal effectively with caregiving problems will save you time in the end.

- Concentrate on positive thoughts. Caregivers who say, "I look for the silver lining," or "I count my blessings and appreciate what my spouse can still do" report that they feel less burdened.

- Relying on religious or philosophical beliefs to help accept the illness and its consequences on their life reduces the burden for some caregivers.

*What patient behaviors and habits contribute to perceived burden?*

- Repeatedly asking questions.

- Constant clinging because of a need to be physically near the caregiver

- Confusion

- Aggression

- Nighttime wandering

*What can I do if these burdens weigh heavily on me?*

- Develop good communications skills with your patient to help eliminate repetitive questions. (See Chapter 3)

- Allow your patient to spend time with other family members. It will help your patient break that strong emotional attachment to you. If other family members are not available, an adult day care setting may be helpful in easing separation anxiety for your patient. The more people in your patient's life, the less complete his or her dependency and attachment to you will be.

- Use humor to lighten the burden when these stressors occur. Research shows that a healthy sense of humor relieves caregiver burden.

## How Stress Affects the Lives of Caregivers

The results of stress can affect caregivers in many ways. Some caregivers find their physical and mental well being is under attack. Anxiety, depression, a diminished social life, and a loss of self-esteem are some of the problems with which caregivers struggle.

Caregivers are always time-starved. But when you order your list of priorities remember that stress-relieving activities should be near the top of your "To Do" list.

### What problems cause the most anxiety for the caregiver?

- Physical and emotional strain of attending to a patient's activities of daily living.

- Keeping a patient out of harm's way.

- Managing difficult patient behavior such as agitation and wandering.

- Conflicts with other family members.

- Limitations on personal leisure and social activities.

### How can I relieve the anxiety of caregiving?

If you are the lone caregiver, it may be difficult to find time for yourself. But it is vital to your emotional health.

- If no family member or friend is available to stay with your patient occasionally, consider adult day care on a part-time basis. Use the free time to restore your emotional well being. Don't feel guilty about your time away from your patient. You've earned it!

- Take a walk in the sunshine.

- Take an evening stroll.

- Take care of your friendships. Allow your friends to help. Often, we don't realize that friends feel powerless to lighten our burden. They actually are relieved when we suggest something specific that they can do to help.

- Call your friends. They may stop calling you because they think you don't have time to talk. Make the time.

- Form new friendships with support group members. Visit with them outside of meetings.

- Keep up with your hobbies. They will refresh your mind and spirit. If old hobbies won't fit into your schedule, develop new ones that are less time consuming.

- Don't give up special pleasures such as listening to favorite music, reading, or baking special treats for your family and friends.

- Go to the movies – even it you have to bring the theater to your home with a rented video. Watch the movie while someone else is taking care of your patient. Don't try to grab bits and pieces of it between caregiving duties. That will probably increase anxiety.

### How does the stress of caregiving affect social activities for caregivers and their families?

- Caregivers often lose social contact with friends, members of their house of worship and co-workers. These are the very people we often turn to in times of emotional trouble.

- Caring for a parent has an impact on the life of a married child. Far less time is spent with their spouse. Family members of caregiving children resent the lack of privacy and companionship brought into their lives by an Alzheimer patient.

- Vacations are limited or non-existent for caregivers.

### How important is it to keep my social life healthy?

- If you are a caregiver spouse, the emotional benefits from taking care of your friendships and support systems will give you strength. That reaps benefits for your patient as well.

- If you are caregiver to a parent, it is essential that your family's social life doesn't suffer. For a husband and wife, the health of their marriage needs nurturing also. It is a big challenge, but one that the whole family needs to work toward maintaining.

- If you are single without the responsibilities of child rearing, don't fall into the trap of thinking that you have to be the sole caregiver because you are the one with no spouse and/or children to care for. You are just as entitled to a social life. It is equally important to your emotional good health.

*How does stress affect the self-esteem of caregivers?*

- Caregivers often expect much more from themselves than they can accomplish. They want everything to be done to the best of their ability. When this often-impossible goal is set, self-esteem suffers when the goal cannot be met.

- The caregiver's self-esteem can also suffer because the caregiving role restricts social contact. Social contact bolsters self-esteem. When contact with others is lessened, we value ourselves less. With the loss of self-esteem, feelings of depression may follow.

*Do caregivers develop negative health behaviors?*

Many caregivers adopt such negative health behavior as not exercising regularly or overeating. Smokers may increase the number of cigarettes they smoke each day.

Regular exercise is important for caregivers since it can help reduce stress. Caregivers who exercise regularly show less depression, anxiety, anger, perceived stress and generally have lower blood pressure than caregivers who do not exercise.

*What kinds of exercise can a busy caregiver do?*

- Swimming is an excellent exercise. Consider joining the YMCA or a facility that has flexible pool hours. Then you won't feel pressured to exercise on a time schedule that may not work for you.

- Do breathing exercises. You can do them anywhere. Sit in a comfortable chair with your back straight, but relaxed. Close your eyes; then inhale a deep breath of air. Hold it for 8 to 10 seconds; then slowly exhale. Repeat this procedure whenever you have a few moments. This simple exercise has a calming effect on the nervous system.

- Learn yoga. Most libraries now offer educational videotapes on the many levels of yoga. Start with a beginner's program. Borrowing a variety of yoga tapes is also helpful before you decide to purchase the one that is just right for you.

- Go for a bike ride. If you need solitude, go alone. If not, invite a companion.

- Walking offers many benefits beyond exercise. You can walk with your patient to stimulate his or her mind. Walk with a friend to socialize. Walk with a spouse or child to share a private conversation.

*If overeating becomes a problem, what can I do?*

Eating a balanced diet may seem too obvious to mention. But stress and time constraints are enemies of good nutrition. This is an area where family members or friends can help. Ask them to prepare nutritious casseroles that can be cut and frozen for later use. Having these meals handy can cut down on the temptation to eat fast foods or prepackaged products high in calories, fat, and sodium.

- Get enough rest. Starting your day in an irritable mood can create exactly the type of tension that makes people pick mindlessly at food throughout the day.

- Start your day with breakfast – even if you don't like breakfast! Countless studies have shown that many overweight people are breakfast-skippers.

- Make an effort to eat nutritiously. If your day is so busy that you lose track of what and when you eat, keep a journal handy. Every time you pop some food into your mouth, write it down. If you are gaining weight, this will show you where the culprit is hiding.

- Limit salt and caffeine intake. Salt can cause fluid retention and fluid retention can cause headaches, which may make you irritable. Caffeine can make you edgy and more easily irritated by the demands of caregiving. Regardless of the origin of your irritability, be careful that it doesn't result in overeating as a coping method.

- Drink plenty of water throughout the day. A glass of water right before a meal will help you feel full faster.

- Sit down for meals. Eating on the run results in a less-than-satisfied feeling of fullness.

- Keep plenty of raw, cleaned vegetables handy for a quick snack when hunger strikes.

- If you find that you are relying on prepackaged meals, read the labels closely for calorie, fat, and sodium content.

### *If increased cigarette smoking becomes a problem, what can I do?*

It would be best if you quit smoking altogether. But a more realistic goal is to keep cigarette smoking to a minimum.

- Stress often causes smokers to reach for a cigarette more often than usual. Keep a count of the number of cigarettes you are smoking. If it is increasing, make a conscious effort to cut down.

- Keep a journal or log of when you reach for a cigarette. See if you can reduce the stress associated with those times or consciously say that you will not have a cigarette now, even if you are stressed out at the moment.

- Try a nicotine patch or gum. Even if you've tried these before, there's no harm in trying again.

## How Caregiving Affects Your
## Mental and Physical Health

Surprisingly, Alzheimer caregivers seem to maintain their health fairly well despite the enormous stress they work under. However, the burden of caregiving and its related coping methods can lead to or aggravate certain conditions. In particular, Alzheimer caregivers are especially vulnerable to depression-related insomnia, diabetes, which may develop from poor eating habits, and stress-related hypertension. Finding ways to reduce stress and anxiety can go a long way to help prevent or reduce the severity of many of these problems.

*What types of body complaints do caregivers express?*

Caregivers express a myriad of body complaints. The most common are listed below in order of prevalence.

- Insomnia*
- Headaches
- Excessive perspiration
- Heart palpations
- Bad dreams
  *(Insomnia is by far the number one complaint with 70% of women and almost 50% of men reporting this problem.)

*What can I do to prevent these problems?*

- First, have your physician determine that these problems are not caused by a physical condition.

- Make it a priority to try the solutions offered in this book since these symptoms can all be related to stress and anxiety. Being a relaxed caregiver will benefit your patient and keep you healthy in the process.

*Does alcohol and drug use increase among caregivers?*

Caregivers tend to drink more alcohol than non-caregivers. They also tend to use psychotropic drugs such as those that induce sleep or relaxation, although not to excess. As with everything else, moderation is the key.

*A note of caution: A potentially serious problem can arise when alcohol is combined with a relaxant drug. Consult your physician before combining alcohol with any medication.*

*Do caregivers get enough "quality" sleep?*

- Although the number of hours spent sleeping is not dramatically different, the quality of sleep may be less for caregivers, especially if they use sleep-inducing medications. Drug-induced sleep is not as nourishing to the body as sleep that comes naturally.

*How can I get a good night's sleep without using sleep medications?*

- Limit your caffeine intake, especially after 4 p.m. Replace regular coffee with decaf. Don't forget that caffeine is present in tea and many carbonated beverages. Use the decaffeinated varieties.

- Perform stressful caregiving activities early in the day. Tension at bedtime interferes with your ability to fall or stay asleep.

- Get your patient "tucked in" early enough so that you have time to yourself before you go to bed. You can use that time to unwind from the day's activities.

- If your patient is an early riser, allow enough hours of sleep for yourself by gradually going to bed earlier each evening.

*Is hypertension a risk for caregivers?*

- Anxiety levels are associated with an increase in blood pressure. If anxiety is present in the caregiver-patient relationship, it can result in a rise in blood pressure.

*What can I do to avoid hypertension?*

- Although some people are prone to hypertension, the risk can be modified. Caregivers with the most social contacts have the smallest rise in blood pressure (without considering other contributing health factors).

- Seek your physician's advice if hypertension becomes or remains a problem. It may be necessary to take medications for the condition.

- Keep your weight down, cut back on salt intake, and eat healthy foods. These measures may decrease your blood pressure.

*Is diabetes aggravated by the stress of caregiving?*

Yes, diabetes is aggravated by the stress of caregiving. During periods of stress, high levels of insulin are present in the bloodstream. Insulin normally binds to cells and increases the entry of sugar inside cells where it is used for fuel. Thus, insulin that floats in the bloodstream during stress is less efficient. There are some gender differences in susceptibility to stress-related diabetes.

- Female caregivers who report both a high number of caregiving hassles and who feel anger and hostility have higher insulin levels in their bloodstream.

- Male caregivers often have elevated blood insulin with a high number of daily caregiving hassles. But feelings of anger do not seem to raise insulin levels in men as much as with female caregivers.

These findings indicate that diabetic caregivers need to seek ways to release stress and stay as calm as possible. They should try to understand the causes of and ways to control their anger.

### Is the immune system affected by the stress of caregiving?

Caregivers are especially prone to disorders of the immune system. The main defenders in our immune system are lymphocytes and natural killer cells. Natural killer cells are particularly important in fighting viruses. Stress can lower the activity of natural killer cells.

### What are the consequences of a suppressed immune system?

When natural killer cells fail to suppress a virus in the bloodstream, the virus becomes detectable by the presence of raised antibodies.

- Alzheimer caregivers have raised levels of blood antibodies to both the Epstein-Barr virus, which causes extreme fatigue and the HSV-1 virus that causes cold sores.

- In general, caregivers are more prone to colds and infections because of deficient immune responses.

### What can I do to stay healthy?

- Stay physically fit. Get enough rest, eat a balanced diet, and exercise whenever possible. Learn stress-relieving techniques like yoga and meditation.

- Find simple ways to relax. If you are the primary caregiver, take a long bath when someone else can be with your patient.

- Plan regularly scheduled time-outs. Occasionally arrange a day just for you. If you don't have someone to fill in at home, find out about adult day care in your area. Take that day to do whatever relaxes you most – go shopping and buy something just for you, treat yourself to lunch at a restaurant, or get a massage. Remember, you've earned it!

- Consider respite care for your patient. Take a vacation, no matter how short. Get away from home. A change of scenery can be restorative to your emotional health.

# ZARIT BURDEN INTERVIEW

Circle the response that best describes how you feel:

| | Never | Rarely | Sometimes | Quite Frequently | Nearly Always |
|---|---|---|---|---|---|
| 1. Do you feel that your relative asks for more help than he/she needs? | 0 | 1 | 2 | 3 | 4 |
| 2. Do you feel that because of the time you spend with your relative that you don't have enough time for yourself? | 0 | 1 | 2 | 3 | 4 |
| 3. Do you feel stressed between caring for your relative and trying to meet other responsibilities for your family or work? | 0 | 1 | 2 | 3 | 4 |
| 4. Do you feel embarrassed over your relative's behavior? | 0 | 1 | 2 | 3 | 4 |
| 5. Do you feel angry when you are around your relative? | 0 | 1 | 2 | 3 | 4 |
| 6. Do you feel that your relative currently affects your relationships with other family members or friends in a negative way? | 0 | 1 | 2 | 3 | 4 |
| 7. Are you afraid what the future holds for your relative? | 0 | 1 | 2 | 3 | 4 |
| 8. Do you feel your relative is dependent on you? | 0 | 1 | 2 | 3 | 4 |
| 9. Do you feel strained when you are around your relative? | 0 | 1 | 2 | 3 | 4 |
| 10. Do you feel your health has suffered because of your involvement with your relative? | 0 | 1 | 2 | 3 | 4 |
| 11. Do you feel that you don't have as much privacy as you would like because of your relative? | 0 | 1 | 2 | 3 | 4 |

*continued next page*

# ZARIT BURDEN INTERVIEW continued

|  | Never | Rarely | Sometimes | Quite Frequently | Nearly Always |
|---|---|---|---|---|---|
| 12. Do you feel that your social life has suffered because you are caring for your relative? | 0 | 1 | 2 | 3 | 4 |
| 13. Do you feel uncomfortable about having friends over because of your relative? | 0 | 1 | 2 | 3 | 4 |
| 14. Do you feel that your relative seems to expect you to take care of him/her as if you were the only one he/she could depend on? | 0 | 1 | 2 | 3 | 4 |
| 15. Do you feel that you don't have enough money to take care of your relative in addition to the rest of your expenses? | 0 | 1 | 2 | 3 | 4 |
| 16. Do you feel that you will be unable to take care of your relative much longer? | 0 | 1 | 2 | 3 | 4 |
| 17. Do you feel you have lost control of your life since your relative's illness? | 0 | 1 | 2 | 3 | 4 |
| 18. Do you wish you could leave the care of your relative to someone else? | 0 | 1 | 2 | 3 | 4 |
| 19. Do you feel uncertain about what to do about your relative? | 0 | 1 | 2 | 3 | 4 |
| 20. Do you feel you should be doing more for your relative? | 0 | 1 | 2 | 3 | 4 |
| 21. Do you feel you could do a better job in caring for your relative? | 0 | 1 | 2 | 3 | 4 |
| 22. Overall, how burdened do you feel in caring for your relative? | 0 | 1 | 2 | 3 | 4 |

## How to Score the Zarit Burden Interview:

Score 4 for each "nearly always" circled
Score 3 for each "quite frequently" circled
Score 2 for each "sometimes" circled
Score 1 for each "rarely" circled
Score 0 for each "never" circled
Add all the points – possible scores for the test range from 0 to 88, with 88 being the greatest possible burden.

## Test Results:

Based on total score, you are experiencing the following degree of caregiver burden:
0-20 = little or no burden
21-40 = mild to moderate burden
41-60 = moderate to severe burden
61-88 = severe burden

*The Zarit Burden Interview is used with the permission of Steven H. Zarit, Ph.D.*

*Chapter Topics and Suggested Readings*
*from the Alzheimer's Association 2001 Public Publications Catalog:*

Caregiver Stress: Signs to Watch for ... Steps to Take – brochure
Managing Difficult Behavior – VHS video
Adult Day Care – fact sheet
Are You a Healthy Caregiver – fact sheet
Especially for the Alzheimer Caregiver (how to cope with caregiving) – brochure
Meeting Daily Challenges (strategies for structuring a daily schedule) – VHS video
Respite Care Guide (recognizing the benefits of respite care) – guide
You Can Make a Difference: 10 Ways to Help an Alzheimer Family – a brochure

# Chapter Eight

## Sources of Support
## for
## The Caregiver

~ *" We all of us need assistance.*
*Those who sustain others themselves*
*want to be sustained"* ~

Maurice Hulst

## Support Groups—
## Are They Right For You?

Support groups for family members and caregivers became more prevalent after the National Alzheimer's Association was formed in 1980. Today, many hospitals, educational institutions, religious organizations, and government social service agencies also sponsor support groups for Alzheimer caregivers. These groups range in size from a few people meeting informally to discuss problems to large, formal organizations. Check with your local or county government agency, newspapers, libraries, and the Alzheimer's Association at 800-272-3900 for contact numbers. Your family physician may also have support group information.

Timing is important. Caregiver needs change as the disease progresses. Join a group when you are ready. Don't hesitate to shop around until you find a group that is a comfortable fit for your needs and temperament.

### Who attends Alzheimer support groups?

- About 75% of all caregivers belong to a support group.

- Support group members are primarily women between the ages of 40 to 65.

- Most group members care for patients in the moderate to severe dementia range.

### What happens at a support group meeting?

- Groups generally meet once a month for 1 to 2 hours.

- They are led by a trained leader, often a social worker, nurse, or psychologist.

- Typical activities of a group session include: discussion of problems or ideas, presentation of formal education about dementia, introduction of new members, socializing, guest speakers, and resource information and referral.

### What do members like best about support groups?

- Meeting others with similar concerns

- Finding out how others deal with problems

- Gaining a better understanding of Alzheimer's disease

- Sharing feelings with other members

- Feeling less isolated and alone

90

- Obtaining information about health and social services

- Gaining information about legal and financial resources

- Gaining a better sense of competence as a caregiver

- Learning new caregiving skills

- Reducing guilt feelings and coping with personal anger

- Learning to enhance relations with the care recipient

- Coping with fears for the future

- Learning how to get along with other family members

### *Are there certain aspects of support groups that some caregivers don't like?*

- Sometimes members feel drained by each other rather than supported by one another.

- The business of fundraising and advocacy can provide additional stress to an already overstressed caregiver.

### *Does attending a support group help caregivers?*

- Numerous studies have shown that regular attendance does decrease caregiver burden.

- Findings are less clear and somewhat conflicting about whether support groups decrease depression and anxiety for the caregiver. Although support groups do not make *major* changes in depression or feelings of perceived caregiving burden, caregivers do find the groups valuable for other reasons. In the end, the caregiver must decide whether the time spent at support group meetings is time well spent.

### *How can I start my own support group?*

If you can't find a group that fits your needs, start your own.

- Advertise locally in newspapers, religious and community organization bulletin boards, or your local library for other interested caregivers.

- Ask your family physician, nurse practitioner, or social worker for advice on forming a group.

- Prepare information about frequency of meetings, times, and location.

Consider using a town hall or library meeting room so that no one has the responsibility of acting as host or hostess.

- Let potential members know that membership is free of charge.

- Clarify your criteria for membership. For example, decide if you want an age limit or if teens and children can be included.

When your group is formed, explain that every member should honor the confidentiality of any discussions taking place at meetings. This agreement will help create an open atmosphere where members feel free to discuss sensitive issues.

# Support Professionals and Home Health Aides

Professional sources of support and home health aides provide valuable relief to the burden of caregiving. Your healthcare team can step in if you become ill or temporarily unavailable for your patient. They can perform some of the chores you would rather delegate such as housekeeping or personal grooming for your patient. Then you can focus on the skills you bring to caregiving.

If paying for these services is more than you can afford, check out sources of support and financial aid mentioned in Appendix B. You may qualify for subsidized support.

## What kind of professional healthcare support is available to me?

- Registered Nurses (RN) and Licensed Practical Nurses (LPN), if your patient has special medical needs in addition to Alzheimer's.

- Medical social workers – They evaluate patient and caregiver needs, make referrals, and provide counseling.

- Physical and occupational therapists.

- Home health aides – Usually provide personal patient care. They can help with direct care needs such as meals, medications, transportation of your patient, and supervision of your patient when you need to be away from home.

## Where can I find information on how to obtain services?

The Visiting Nurse Associations of America (VNAA) is the official, national association of freestanding not-for-profit, community-based visiting nurse agencies. You can find a member Visiting Nurse Agency located near you by contacting the national organization.

## How can I contact the Visiting Nurse Associations?

- Visit their website at **www.vnaa.org**

- Call them at 617-523-4042

- Contact them by mail at: 11 Beacon St., Suite 910, Boston, MA 02108

*Can I learn about financial support for home health care from the VNAA?*

Yes. If you visit the website, go to "Caregiver Information – Commonly Asked Questions". You will find a discussion under "Will my insurance cover home healthcare?" Or call the VNAA. The website also provides a listing of all local Visiting Nurse Association members by state.

*What other kind of help is available?*

Nurses' aides, homemakers, or care providers can help supervise and provide personal care for your patient. They also can help with your housekeeping chores to allow you more time with your patient.

# Community Services
## When to Use Them, How to Find Them

Community resources allow family members to care for their patient without placing severe limitations on their own lives. Even if you don't need these resources in the early stages of caregiving, learn about them. As demands on your time and energy grow, community services will become more important. They can reduce the physical and mental strain on you and your patient.

*What types of community services do most caregivers want?*

- Respite care (adult day & overnight care)

- Personal or nursing care

- Caregiver education

- Financial and legal assistance

- Meal preparation services

- Home modification

- Housework assistance

*How can I locate community services in my area?*

- Contact the Alzheimer's Association, which has chapters throughout the United States and knows what services are available locally for Alzheimer caregivers. The organization can be reached toll-free at 1-800-272-3900.

- Contact your local area Office of Aging. Many county governments in the United States have these agencies. The agencies offer information about community resources for caregivers and senior citizens. Consult the white pages or local government pages of your telephone directory for contact numbers. Your local library may also keep lists of available services.

*Respite Care*
*What's Available*
*Does It Relieve Caregiver Burden?*

The challenges facing caregivers can be unrelenting. Seeking support from outside sources often brings relief to overburdened caregivers. Family members need a break from the continuous care required of their patient. Caregivers under constant emotional stress can greatly benefit from respite programs.

Respite at nursing homes can offer caregivers a safe haven for their patient in times of crisis. Certain situations such as the development of serious behavior problems, or an injury sustained by the patient may not be severe enough to qualify for hospitalization. But these problems may need more attention than the caregiver can supply either physically or emotionally. Nursing home respite is an alternative to consider.

This chapter discusses avenues beyond the family to help lighten the load many caregivers carry throughout the long goodbye.

### What is respite?

Respite care is the most widely used form of community service. Respite is a broad term that may include:

- Temporary nursing home placement

- Home health care

- Home companions

- Adult day care

### What types of respite are available? When will respite care help?

### Temporary nursing home placement

- May become necessary if your patient sustains an injury. Once the patient has received hospital treatment, he or she may need to recuperate and receive rehabilitation from either a physical or occupational therapist. Such treatment can be administered during a short nursing home stay.

- Many nursing homes accept Alzheimer patients for a short stay if the caregiver needs to be away or is going away on vacation.

- Some nursing homes also accept patients who have been hospitalized for serious behavior problems once they have been evaluated and stabilized with medications.

You may have to pay for respite care in a nursing home with your own or your patient's funds, depending on the reason for the patient's stay. Whether your patient will qualify for Medicaid payment of these types of nursing home stays depends upon evaluation by Medicaid representatives. Always check with nursing home administrators about fees you will incur for temporary nursing home stays. Generally, they can tell you whom to contact about insurance coverage.

## Home Day Care

- Supervision and personal care are important but demanding needs for an Alzheimer patient. Some patients must be watched vigilantly, especially if they wander. A primary caregiver functions under tremendous pressure while trying to accomplish all the many chores required caring for a home and family as well as a patient. Guarding against physical fatigue and the emotional breakdown of a caregiver makes home health care extremely important.

- Whether the home day care provider is a healthcare professional or an aide depends on the needs of the patient and caregiver. In the earlier stages of Alzheimer's, a healthcare professional is not needed unless the patient has a coexisting medical problem.

## Adult Day Care

Caregivers live in a variety of family situations. Many cannot afford to stay at home with their patient because they need income from their job. Also, not every person who finds himself or herself in the role of caregiver is suited for that responsibility. Many reasons exist for placing a patient in adult day care.

If family members feel confident about the place their loved one will spend a portion of each day, then the guilt that often accompanies this decision can be relieved.

- Adult day care provides a safe environment for the patient during the caregiver's working hours.

- Day care provides patients with a scheduled routine of exercise, recreation, stimulating activities, and socialization with other patients.

- Some facilities provide social workers, nurses, physical and occupational therapists.

- Schedules vary at most adult day care centers. Some accept patients on an "as needed" basis. This can provide great comfort to harried caregivers or for those who need temporary supervision for their patient.

- For patients who do not attend adult day care, it can be vital to have a place available if an emergency arises. Knowing that there is safe shelter for a loved one, if suddenly needed, can provide you with peace of mind.

*A note of caution: make sure that the adult day care facility you choose handles patients with cognitive and behavior problems. Many senior citizen centers are not equipped to handle such problems.*

One valuable aspect of respite care is that it frequently allows decisions for nursing home placement to be delayed. Making a nursing home decision is one of the most difficult of Alzheimer caregiving. When families cope more effectively with caregiver burden, they often postpone nursing home placement. When a patient reaches a severe stage of dementia, and caregivers know and accept that there is no alternative, it becomes a more peaceful decision for everyone involved.

# Other Sources of Support
## Family, Friends, Spiritual Guidance, Pets

The tremendous burden and responsibility of caring for an Alzheimer patient is often too much for one person to shoulder. Even though some caregivers try to go it alone, help from other sources may not only help to ease your burden, but with compassion and understanding, perhaps even bring family and friends closer together during a most stressful life passage.

*Does strong support from within a caregiver's family relieve caregiver burden?*

Support from a close-knit family is very helpful for caregivers. Numerous studies have established that strong family support dramatically reduces caregiver burden.

*What kind of family support helps caregivers most?*

- Providing respite care (staying with the patient so the caregiver can leave home for a while)

- Visiting the caregiver, not just the patient

- Preparing a meal

- Cooking or cleaning

- Arranging appointments

- Accompanying the patient to the doctor

- Providing physical care for the patient

- Handling legal and business matters

*Does family support have drawbacks?*

Yes. The intensity of Alzheimer caregiving creates an emotionally charged atmosphere among family members as their lives become more intertwined.

- Conflict often arises over complaints that siblings fail to help as much as they should.

- Serious conflicts often arise with other family members about how to provide care for the patient.

## How can I avoid or limit conflict among my family members?

- Be alert to early signs of conflict. Deal with problems as they arise. Don't let problems simmer to the boiling point.

- Keep an open dialogue among family members. Suggest a family meeting occasionally, and allow each member to speak freely about feelings.

- If the conflict escalates, consult a family counselor.

## What will a strong social network do for a caregiver?

A large social network with many friends and acquaintances significantly lowers caregiver depression and burden. No matter how busy you are, don't lose contact with friends.

- Caregivers with a large circle of friends have better health than caregivers with only a few friends.

- Alzheimer caregivers with a large social circle tend to have lower blood pressure when under stress than caregivers without a strong social circle.

- Sharing a laugh with friends is beneficial. Maintaining a sense of humor will help you maintain your emotional health. And emotional good health reduces stress and its accompanying physical problems.

- Friends want to help and feel much better if they can do something to lighten your burden. Allow them to give you support. Both of you will benefit.

- Taking a friend or group of friends along for a walk or a bike ride not only gives you a chance to socialize, but you get the benefits of exercise.

- Maintaining a social life with your circle of friends will force you to get away from your caregiving role occasionally. Honoring yourself is essential to keeping your mental health in good shape. Friends help you remember who you are.

## Does attending religious services help ease caregiver burden?

Regularly attending services at a house of worship can reduce caregiver burden. One study showed that attending religious services on a regular basis was the strongest predictor of psychological well being.

## Why is attending religious services so beneficial to caregivers?

- Religious services provide spiritual and inspirational support. Our religious belief systems often help us accept the burdens we must bear.

- Speaking privately with the spiritual leader of your religious affiliation can bring comfort and reduce caregiver burden.

- Support systems for those in need are already in place in houses of worship.

- Being with other members of a religious group provides caregivers with the chance to socialize. Socializing is an important way to relieve caregiver burden.

If attending religious services creates anxiety or agitation in your patient, find a way to continue attending without your patient. The benefits are too great to give up. Consult members of your religious affiliation's support system to see if respite is available during services.

### Do pets help ease caregiver burden?

Although countless studies have shown that living with a pet reduces blood pressure and offers companionship, dealing with the introduction of a new pet can create more of a burden than it relieves. Several important issues should be considered before making a decision about bringing new pets into the home of an Alzheimer patient.

You also will need to take precautions with pets already in your household. Being prepared in advance will help eliminate some of the inevitable problems and resultant burden.

### What can I do if I already have a pet?

- Make sure your pet is confined during the overnight hours, especially if your patient is a wanderer.

- Purchase a kennel. You may need to confine your pet while attending your patient.

- Have a safe room in your home to confine your pet, if it should suddenly become necessary. Keep the door closed rather than using a baby gate, which could be dangerous to an Alzheimer patient.

- Check out pet-sitting services before you need one. Ask if they take pets on short notice.

### Should I get a pet?

The realities of owning a pet, especially a dog or cat, and how strongly a caregiver feels about having a pet will make a significant difference in caregiver burden. If you don't already have a pet, ask yourself the following questions.

- Are you *really* up to assuming the responsibility of full-time pet care? Don't deceive yourself. The responsibility of taking care of a pet is huge and time-consuming.

- If you are alone for long periods of time with your patient, will it be safe to leave your patient unattended to take the pet outside?

- How will your patient respond to a pet? Pets can be very beneficial to soothing an anxious person. But if your patient did not have or like pets before developing Alzheimer's, he or she will be less likely to tolerate them now. You don't want to add to your burden by creating a new problem.

- Will your pet be a hazard to your patient? Small dogs and cats are difficult to see when they are under foot. Patients with limited vision, mobility, and poor balance could easily fall and injure themselves and the pet. If you already own a pet, be very careful when the pet is around your patient. An angry Alzheimer patient may antagonize an otherwise friendly animal.

## Chapter Topics and Suggested Readings
## from the Alzheimer's Association 2001 Public Publications Catalog:

### Support Professionals and Other Health Aides

Know Your Rights to Cure and Treatment in a Nursing Home – guide

### Community Services

Caring in the Community – report
Services You May Need (such as medical, financial, and care services) – fact sheet

### Respite Care

Respite Care Guide – guide
Adult Day Care – fact sheet
Hospitalization – fact sheet

### Other Sources of Support

Caring for the Caregiver (includes how to build networks of support including
        family, friends, and respite services) – VHS video
Holidays – fact sheet
You Can Make a Difference: 10 Ways to Help an Alzheimer Family – brochure
Alzheimer's Disease: A Guide for Clergy – brochure

# Chapter Nine

## The Emotional Aspects
## of
## Caregiving

~ *"Some people weave burlap into the fabric of our lives and*
*some weave gold thread. Both contribute to make the*
*whole picture beautiful and unique"* ~

Anonymous

# *Depression Among Caregivers*

The downward spiral of depression can silently cripple the spirit of a caregiver. Often, caregivers have the best intentions when they decide to "go it alone." They don't ask for help, they quietly slip away from their friends and support systems, and pride may prevent them from seeking financial assistance. Severe emotional and physical problems can easily develop from a deepening depression. Left untreated, depression not only aggravates existing health problems, but it can create new ones as well.

The best way to prevent caregiver burden from becoming depression is to stay in touch with your emotional state. Be honest with yourself. Denial is your enemy. Depression is highly treatable if help is sought early.

This chapter will help you recognize caregiver depression, what causes it, and how to prevent it from overtaking you.

### *Do men or women suffer more from caregiver-related depression?*

- Studies have shown that female caregivers almost always suffer more feelings of depression than male caregivers.

- Women tend to become depressed very early in the caregiving process.

- Male caregivers do not get depressed early on, but by 24 months, their depression scores approach the levels of female caregivers.

### *Why do spouses become more depressed than other family members?*

Spouses usually care for their Alzheimer patient for longer time periods than do other family members. The longer a patient suffers from dementia, the more severe behavior problems become. So it follows, that spouses would be at higher risk for depression.

### *How can I tell if I'm depressed?*

One way you can measure the extent of your depressed feelings is to take the Beck Depression Inventory, invented by Dr. Aaron Beck. This test is widely used to measure the degree of depression from which someone is suffering.

The test is easy to score. If the test indicates mild depression, it is in your best interest to seek medical help to prevent a mild problem from becoming a major problem. If the test reveals that you have significant depression, it is even more important that you seek medical consultation.

You can access the test by using a search engine such as **www.google.com**. Then, type in "Beck Depression Inventory" in the Search box.

*What are some of the physical signs and symptoms of depression?*

- Unexplained fatigue and dizzy spells

- Gastrointestinal problems such as indigestion and constipation

- Changes in eating habits, appetite, and weight (gain or loss)

- Frequently awakening later or earlier than normal, or sleeping disturbances such as waking up during the night

*What are some of the psychological symptoms of depression?*

- Irritability and anxiety

- Loss of interest in friends and social contacts

- Loss of sexual desire

- Feelings of despair, hopelessness, or thoughts of suicide

- Guilt, anger, low self-esteem

- Apathy, restlessness, boredom

- Loss of interest in grooming and personal hygiene

- Loss of interest in favorite activities such as hobbies

*How is depression different than simply "feeling down in the dumps"?*

- Guilt and anger are normal emotions in a caregiving situation. But if an overwhelming sense of hopelessness and despair develop from guilt and anger, you may be experiencing depression.

- Depression is a prolonged disturbance of mood. It changes your perception of the world. If the feeling of hopelessness and despair lasts for more than 2 weeks, you may be depressed.

*What are some causes of depression for Alzheimer caregivers? What can I do to help decrease the risk of depression?*

- The longer number of years spent in the caregiving role, the worse depression becomes. As time goes on, it becomes essential that you ask for hands-on help with your patient.

- The number of hours spent in daily caregiving. Ideally, you need a break *every* day.

- Living in the same home as your patient increases your likelihood of depression. If you live with your patient, avoid slipping into depression by asking other family members to relieve you from caregiving duties whenever possible.

- Those with lower income levels may not have sufficient income to hire outside help for caregiving. Search for free or reduced-fee help if you cannot afford respite care. Start by calling your local or county Office of Aging. (See Appendix B for other sources of financial aid.)

*What patient problems will affect my ability to avoid depression?*

Studies have shown that caregivers are greatly bothered by patients who:

- Are verbally or physically abusive.

- Disrupt meals.

- Fail to cooperate with the caregiver.

- Embarrass the caregiver in front of others.

The depression level of caregivers can rise in relationship to the number and frequency of behavior problems presented by the patient.

*How will my attitude influence depression?*

- Perfectionists and achievement-oriented people are at risk of depression because the caregiving role can prove extremely frustrating to this Type A personality.

- Caregivers who use confrontation to alter situations display more anger and hostility. This magnifies problem behavior in the patient, which in turn contributes to caregiver depression.

*How can I handle anger if my patient is difficult?*

- See the section of Chapter 3 that discusses dealing with caregiver anger.

- Try relaxation techniques such as deep breathing.

- Respond, rather than react, to situations. That adage, "Count to 10 before you say anything," just might help.

*Do most caregivers seek treatment for depression?*

Only about one-third of caregivers seek adequate medical help for their depression. Why?

- Because they don't realize they are depressed. Assessing your mental health is extremely important. Take the Zarit Burden Interview at the end of Chapter 7 to determine the amount of caregiver burden you are experiencing. Caregiver burden can develop into depression. The Beck Depression Inventory will help to assess your level of depression. See *How can I tell if I'm depressed?* in this chapter to learn how to access The Beck Depression Inventory.

- Caregivers often assume that placement of a loved one in a nursing home will make depression disappear because they will have more free time for leisure activities and socializing.

**Will depression become less of a problem once my patient is placed in a nursing home or has died?**

- While it is true that life becomes easier when a loved one is placed in a nursing home, many studies show that untreated depression is just as serious a problem among these caregivers as among those who have their patient at home.

- Depression can remain at high levels for up to two years after a patient dies. The caregiver's need for continuing professional consultation still exists even after the patient is placed in a nursing home or subsequently dies.

The best way to treat depression is to stop it before it becomes entrenched in your life. Awareness remains your best weapon. *Depression is highly treatable if help is sought early.*

## Sexual Intimacy
## Between Caregiver and Patient

Sexual intimacy and its inherent problems between a caregiver and a loved one is a concern not often addressed. Although this subject is not as openly discussed as other issues at support group meetings, caregivers do discuss specific problems involving sexual intimacy when encouraged.

If you are in a support group and feel comfortable with frank discussions about sexual intimacy issues, tell your group members. Ask them if it is okay to talk about the subject openly. If some members are uncomfortable with this type of discussion, consider setting up a sub-group to talk about sexual intimacy. Or, perhaps interested members can remain after the regular meeting for such discussions.

### What concerns about sexual intimacy distress caregivers?

- Sexual overtures from a spouse who no longer recognizes his or her partner.

- The realization that their spouse cannot remember recently shared intimacy makes some caregivers uncomfortable about sexual relations.

- Patient incontinence and poor personal hygiene may affect the caregiver's sexual desire.

### What are some problems that may hinder intimacy?

Among couples still desiring sexual intimacy, numerous factors can interfere with sexual relations. A few common problems are:

- More than half of all male Alzheimer patients have complete loss of erectile function.

- The patient may forget the sequence of steps involved in lovemaking.

- Caregivers are too tired to feel an interest in sexual intimacy.

- Feelings about initiating sex with a spouse who clearly cannot consent or refuse may cause guilt or embarrassment. This is a special concern of male caregivers.

- Caregiver wives often experience guilt about rejecting the sexual advances of their husbands. They feel that they are not fulfilling their marital vows. And they don't want to hurt their husband's pride.

*How can a caregiver deal with these problems?*

- Do not feel guilty if you no longer desire sexual intimacy with your patient. As in any other sexual relationship, it should be consensual. Touching, hugging, and cuddling can ease the loss of the physical act of lovemaking. Spending time in close physical proximity to one another can help fulfill the need for intimacy.

- Accept that eventually the sex drive of the Alzheimer patient will diminish substantially or disappear due to the nature of the disease. Don't take this as a personal affront to your desirability.

- Discuss the pain and loneliness that comes with changes in your patient's sexual behavior. Talking with close family members, friends, or support group members can help ease this transition in your relationship.

*Is dementia the cause of change in sexual activity in Alzheimer's?*

Yes. Changes in sexual activity are common in many dementing diseases. One kind of dementia is called frontal lobe dementia. More than 50% of frontal lobe dementia sufferers lose interest in sexual activity. Even though the frontal lobe of Alzheimer patients is less affected than in other forms of dementia, the same symptoms may be present.

*What happens to the relationship once sex becomes a thing of the past?*

- Once active sexual relations ends, it is likely that you will spend more time holding hands or hugging. The sense of touch remains well preserved in many patients, even in advanced stages of the disease. *Touch is a special gift we never seem to lose.*

- How a couple touches one another is often altered by caregiving. Studies show that Alzheimer couples spend more time holding hands or patting the other on the shoulder. The interplay between Alzheimer patients and caregivers heightens the use of touch.

*Will I experience any particularly difficult sexual behavior by my patient? What can I do?*

- As the disease progresses, patients may touch themselves inappropriately or even expose themselves. Although this is disturbing, try to remember that your patient has forgotten the rules of etiquette. You will have to remind your patient each time an incident occurs since he or she will not remember the previous incident.

- If your patient has become paranoid, he or she may accuse you of sexual misbehavior. Simply seeing you with another person may be enough to cause suspicion. Remember that paranoid behavior doesn't respond to reason or argument. A little extra touching, hugging, or stroking of your patient may help calm the situation. But don't force physical contact if your patient clearly does not want to be touched.

*What are some common misconceptions about inappropriate sexual behavior that I might encounter?*

Many people have the view that those suffering from dementia constantly engage in sexual activity and exhibitionism. Is there any truth to that belief?

- Only a small percentage of demented patients ever display a sexually inappropriate behavior. When these behaviors occur, they are usually brief and mild.

- At times what appears to be blatant sexual exhibitionism may not be. For example, an Alzheimer patient appearing in public incompletely dressed is not necessarily a form of sexual exhibitionism. Most of these patients are simply unable to dress themselves properly and nothing of a sexual nature is intended.

- The patient may become too warm or uncomfortable and begin to remove articles of clothing in public. Patients forget what they once knew about modesty.

- Alzheimer's disease can cause repetitive motions and fidgeting such as playing with buttons and zippers. This could be misconstrued as sexual in nature.

# Violence
## The Hidden Problem Among
### Caregivers and Patients

Violence in a caregiver-care recipient relationship is rarely addressed as a caregiving issue. Because violence is not discussed openly, it is difficult to know to what extent this potentially serious situation occurs. Caregivers may be reluctant to report an act of violence by their patient because they fear what will happen once the police are called. But you can take comfort in the fact that there is an increased awareness of the behavior of Alzheimer patients by members of the law enforcement community in our country.

Many members of police departments in America are taking part in sensitivity training either from their own personnel, other law enforcement agencies, or from training offered by the National Alzheimer's Association through local chapters across the country. Law enforcement officers are learning how to deal effectively and compassionately with Alzheimer patients who have become violent.

As in most situations involving Alzheimer's disease, it falls upon caregivers to assume responsibility to safeguard both themselves and their patient against anger and violence.

*(A personal note from Jim Knittweis: On the few occasions when it became necessary to ask the police to assist us with my father's aggressive or violent behavior, the police officers involved handled the situation with gentleness and compassion.)*

### How common is violence by the patient toward the caregiver?

- More than half of caregivers have experienced some kind of violence from their patient.

- It is more frequent than violence from caregivers toward patients.

- Patients who are violent tend to be repeatedly violent.

- Violence by patients toward caregivers is one reason caregivers decide to admit their patient to a nursing home.

### What diminished mental capacities of a patient result in violent behavior?

- Hallucinations caused by sensory impairment may result in misinterpretation of sights and sounds and can cause a patient to become highly agitated and delusional.

- Delusions, which are persistent incorrect beliefs despite rational evidence to the contrary, may cause your patient to angrily accuse you of stealing something even when you show the patient the item in dispute.

- Paranoia, very intense suspiciousness, may develop as your patient's interpretation of information and reasoning capabilities diminish. Paranoia can frequently result in violent behavior.

- Catastrophic reaction, a panicked reaction to the events taking place, can cause your patient's mood to change very quickly. He or she may lash out verbally or physically, become combative, or begin to cry inconsolably.

All of these problems can lead from agitation to aggression and violence.

*What are some of the causes of patient violence?*

- Gender plays a role. Male Alzheimer patients are almost twice as likely to be more aggressive than women patients.

- The precursor to violence is aggressiveness. More than half of all Alzheimer patients demonstrate some kind of verbal or physical aggressiveness from time to time.

- The most common situation that creates aggressive behavior in a patient seems to be when the caregiver tells the patient to do something in a demanding tone or in a manner that confuses the patient.

*What types of violent or aggressive behavior do Alzheimer patients display?*

- Physical acts of violence can include pinching, hitting, kicking, shoving, and pushing. Although these may seem minor, they should always be discouraged in a non-confrontational manner.

- Sexual aggression does occur, but only rarely-in less than 10% of patients.

*What actions should I take when a potentially violent situation occurs?*

- Eliminate the source of trouble, if possible. For example, your patient may suddenly no longer recognize you as someone familiar and may become agitated by your presence. Remove yourself from the patient's sight, if someone else can stay with the patient. Then try reintroducing yourself.

- Maintain eye contact.

- Speak slowly and softly in a low-pitched voice.

- Approach your patient from his or her front view. Coming from behind a patient can be perceived as a threat.

- Avoid arguing with your patient. Contradiction will only further frustrate the patient.

- Validate your patient's emotions by statements such as, "You seem angry. Is there something I can do to help?"

- Offer comfort. Ask your patient if he or she would like a hug. But don't force physical contact.

- Avoid restraints. Their use could prompt a catastrophic reaction.

- Distract your patient by changing the subject or moving to a different room.

- Use positive instructions such as, "Let's go to the living room." Don't give orders such as, "Leave this room."

### How can I better communicate with my patient to avoid aggressive and violent behavior?

- Clear communication is an important part of preventing aggressiveness. For helpful hints, see the communication skills outlined in Chapter 3 – *Communicating*.

- Learn effective ways to handle aggression. Refer to Chapter 3 – *Managing Anger and Aggression*

### If all else fails, are there drugs available to my help my patient?

- Unfortunately, for many patients the only way to control escalating aggression is with prescription pharmaceutical drugs. Drugs are usually regarded as a last resort measure.

- Until recently, the standard drugs to treat agitation have been haloperidol and thioridazine. While these drugs are effective, they have a high incidence of side effects.

- Risperidone is currently the prescribed drug of choice for agitation in dementia. Consult your physician to determine which drug is best for your patient. If any drugs are causing side effects in your patient, ask your physician about alternative medications. Some minor side effects from medications can be controlled with other medications.

  *Always consult your physician before discontinuing any of your patient's prescription drugs.*

*What causes caregivers to become or fear that they will become violent with their patient?*

- One study found that seriously depressed caregivers are three times more likely to commit violence against their patient.

- Some caregivers fear becoming violent with their patient. Caring for a very impaired Alzheimer patient and struggling with low self-esteem seem to increase this fear. Most often, it is the spouse of a patient who suffers this fear.

*How can I reduce the possibility that I might become violent toward my patient?*

- Be alert to caregiver burden that can lead to depression. Take the Zarit Burden Interview (Chapter 7) and the Beck Depression Inventory (see this chapter – *How can I tell if I'm depressed?*). If they indicate that you may be overburdened or depressed, seek professional counseling.

- When you feel overwrought by caregiving, find respite care for your patient. (See Chapter 8 – *Respite Care*)

- Talk with your health care provider if you fear that caregiver violence may become a problem for you.

# Caregiver Grief –
## "The Funeral That Never Ends"

Caring for a relative with Alzheimer's disease has been described as the "funeral that never ends." Caregivers see their loved one dying a little each day, gradually becoming a shadow of the person they once were.

There is no denying that this is a difficult emotional journey. You will need to call on your inner strength. Accepting the disease's presence in your life will help make the emotional and physical strains on you, your patient, and your family a little less overwhelming.

Grieving will be an ongoing process while your patient is alive and will continue after your patient dies. Although many caregivers feel a temporary sense of relief upon the death of the loved one, common feelings at the time of death can include depression, a yearning for the deceased, and a flood of memories. With the passage of time and support, peace and acceptance will come.

***As a caregiver, what stages of grief will I most likely experience during my patient's illness?***

Because Alzheimer's involves a lingering death, the stages of grief are very similar to the stages of adjustment to impending death described by Elizabeth Kubler-Ross in her 1969 book, *On Death and Dying.* Five general stages of grief were identified. But not every caregiver experiences these stages in the same way or for the same length of time. Keep that in mind as you read the following.

**Stage One –** *Denial*
> Denial is usually experienced at the time Alzheimer's is first diagnosed. Family members and the eventual caregiver do not believe the diagnosis. They want to believe that the doctor is mistaken. Often, they seek a second opinion – sometimes a third. Others simply ignore the diagnosis and pretend that everything will be fine.

**Stage Two –** *Anger and Resentment*
> Anger may be directed at many people – the doctors, other family members, or toward God. Caregivers in this stage may resent their loved one for becoming ill and causing physical, mental, and financial hardships.

**Stage Three –** *Bargaining*
> In this stage, caregivers try to "buy back" their loved one's life with some promise, often to God. They make bargains by saying, "I will do anything if you will bring back my loved one's health." They try to postpone the disease from worsening by searching for new therapies, giving the patient home remedies, or by taking their patient to non-traditional therapists.

### Stage Four – *Depression*

In this stage, the illness and eventual death of the patient is realized as inevitable. Feelings of despair, sleeplessness, social isolation, and physical illness may plague the caregiver.

### Stage Five – *Acceptance*

In the last grief stage, caregivers fully accept the situation and the inevitability of the death of the patient. They live each day as best they can. They relish the thought that their loved one, although impaired, is still with them. They are at peace with what is happening. But it is important to note that for Alzheimer caregivers, this feeling of peace may be short-lived. Some caregivers suffer from depression upon the death of their loved one, but eventually peace and acceptance return.

### *How does guilt and anger affect a caregiver's grief?*

If caregivers feel guilt or anger toward the patient, these feelings can make the caregiver's preparation for their patient's eventual death more difficult. The following are some of the reasons caregivers experience guilt and anger.

- Guilt for placing the loved one in a nursing home. Some caregivers believe that they were not caring enough and perhaps could have done something to prevent a nursing home placement.

- Anger toward the patient who is making their life more difficult.

- Anger with other kin who they believe are not sharing in the caregiving burden.

- Anger at a social system that places economic hardship on the patient and the caregiver.

### *How can I rid myself of so much guilt and anger?*

- Be aware of and acknowledge the existence and validity of your feelings.

- Talk with someone – a spiritual adviser, professional counselor, close friend, or compassionate family member. It will help you release the guilt and anger.

- Don't assume that your relatives know how you feel about their not sharing the burden. Discuss your feelings with them in as calm a way as possible. People often get so caught up in their own lives that they don't realize they are falling short of the responsibilities they should be assuming. Many people believe that if you are not complaining, then everything is all right.

- Discuss your complaints in a controlled setting. For example, set a time and place to air your feelings so that they don't pop out as an angry statement. Make a list of what you want to say and stick to that list.

- Delegate the types of chores that are most comfortable and appropriate to other family members. Offer a few alternatives to each.

- Tell your relatives that if they can't fulfill a specific request, it is okay. But ask them to do something else in place of that request.

- If some family members live out of your area, ask them to help by doing some Internet research for information on how to make life easier for you and your patient. Ask them to check out any social services and sources of financial aid that might be available.

- Don't get angry if someone doesn't come through. Make sure that they haven't forgotten about your request or been delayed for a valid reason.

*What determines the amount of grief caregivers experience when their loved one dies?*

Research has shown the following:

- If a close bond was shared during the illness, then grief is felt less at the time of death. But if there were ambivalent feelings and guilt between the caregiver and care recipient, then the caregiver may feel more grief at the time of death.

- Caregivers who receive support and comfort from family and friends at the time of death seem to feel less grief than caregivers who remain isolated.

- Spouse caregivers who frequently talk with others about the death of their spouse find that they think less often about the spouse's passing a year later.

- Caregivers who place their loved ones in a nursing home experience far greater grief than those caregivers whose loved one dies at home.

- Caregivers who feel the most caregiver burden seem to have the most grief when their patient dies.

*Are there unexpected feelings that caregivers experience immediately after the death of their loved one?*

- A feeling of relief, which is often accompanied by guilt for this feeling.

- A sense that their mourning had taken place for many months before the death. Some caregivers say that they could not cry at the time of their loved one's death but that their most intense crying had been done while performing caregiving duties.

- Feeling that they are ready to let go and get on with life.

*How does the death of a spouse affect caregiver depression?*

- When a very ill spouse dies, the caregiver initially feels a sense of relief from the overwhelming chores of caregiving. For a while, feelings of depression may even diminish. But as months pass after the death, depression actually increases in many caregivers.

- In fact, one study found that about 20% of spouses continued to suffer from major depression for as long as 3 years after the death of their husband or wife.

*How can I prepare for my patient's death to make it less traumatic?*

- Speak openly about this eventuality with other family members. Discussing the details of funeral arrangement with family members while your patient is still alive may be less difficult for you than at the time of death.

- Use these discussions to design a funeral service that will honor what the family believes the patient may have wanted. Since this may take some time to accomplish, it is wise to do your planning while more time is available. Discuss the following:

  - Will your loved one be buried or cremated?

  - Place of burial or scattering of ashes

  - Type of religious service, hymns, music, or readings

  - Headstone or memorial inscriptions

Remember that you can't please all of the people all of the time. Compromise among family members will be necessary.

- Alzheimer patients can suddenly become critically ill. If you see that your loved one is in imminent danger of dying, notify all family members. Give them a chance to say their goodbyes.

- Seek spiritual support. A spiritual adviser can give you the strength and courage to accept your loved one's coming death. He or she may also be a bridge to understanding among distraught family members.

When the end inevitably arrives for a loved one with Alzheimer's, each caregiver has earned the right to grieve in a way that will bring closure and comfort. There are no set rules for grieving. Some want time alone, while others want family members and friends close by. Do what is best for you and take comfort in the noble act you have performed during your journey of the long goodbye.

~ *"… to make an end is to make a beginning. The end is where we start from."* ~
T. S. Eliot

## Chapter Topics and Suggested Readings
## from the Alzheimer's Association 2001 Public Publications Catalog:

*Depression Among Caregivers*

Caregiver Stress: Signs to Watch for … Steps to Take – brochure
You Can Make a Difference: 10 Ways to Help an Alzheimer Family – brochure
How to Be a Long-Distance Caregiver – brochure

*Sexual Intimacy Between Caregiver and Patient*

Sexuality – fact sheet

*Violence – The Hidden Problem Among Caregivers and Patients*

Steps to Understanding Challenging Behavior - brochure
Managing Difficult Behavior – VHS video
Alzheimer's Disease: A Guide for Law Enforcement Officials – guide
Combativeness – fact sheet
Hallucinations – fact sheet
Medications – fact sheet
Drug Research – fact sheet

*Caregiver Grief – "The Funeral That Never Ends"*

Alzheimer's Disease: A Guide for Clergy – brochure
Steps to Facing Late-Stage Care: Making End-of-Life Care Decisions
Ethical Considerations: Issues in Death and Dying – fact sheet
Grief, Mourning, and Guilt – fact sheet
Autopsy: A Lasting Gift for Your Family – brochure

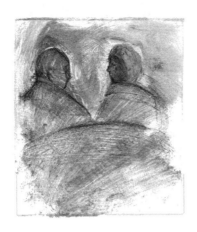

# *Appendix A*

# *Major Alzheimer's Disease Centers*

The National Institute on Aging funds major Alzheimer's Disease Centers
The centers with contact names and numbers are listed by state.

## *Alabama*

University of Alabama at Birmingham
The Sparks Research Center, Suite 454
1720 7th Avenue South
Birmingham AL 35294-0017
Director: Lindy Harrell, M.D., Ph.D.
Director's telephone: 205-934-3847
Information: 205-934-2178
Website: http://main.uab.edu/show.asp?durki=11627

## *California*

Alzheimer's Disease Center
Department of Neurology
University of California, Davis
150 Muir Road (127A)
Martinez CA 94553
Director: William Jagust, M.D.
Director's telephone: 510- 372-2485
Website: http://alzheimer.ucdavis.edu/adc/

Alzheimer's Disease Center
University of California, Los Angeles
710 Westwood Plaza
Los Angeles CA 90095-1769
Director: Jeffrey Cummings, M.D.
Director's telephone: 310-206-5238
Website: http://www.alz.uci.edu/

Alzheimer's Disease Center
Department of Neurosciences
UCSD School of Medicine
9500 Gilman Drive
La Jolla CA 92093-0624
Director: Leon Thal, M.D.
Director's telephone: 858-534-4606
Information: 858-622-5800
Website: http:/adrc.ucsd.edu/

University of Southern California
Andrus Gerontology Center
University Park MC 0191
3715 McClintock Avenue
Los Angeles CA 90089-0191
Co-Director: Caleb Finch, Ph.D.
Director's telephone: 213-740-1758
Co-Director: Carl Cotman, Ph.D.
Director's telephone: 714-824-5847
Information: 213-740-7777
Website: http://www.usc.edu/dept/gero/ADRC/

## Georgia

Emory Alzheimer's Disease Center
Wesley Woods Health Center, 2nd Floor
1841 Clifton Road NE
Atlanta GA 30329
Interim Director: Mahlon DeLong, M.D.
Information: 404-728-6950
Website: http://www.emory.edu/WHSC/MED/ADC

## Illinois

Cognitive Neurology and Alzheimer's Disease Center
Northwestern Medical School
320 East Superior Street, Searle 11-453
Chicago IL 60611
Director: Marsel Mesulam, M.D.
Director's telephone: 312-908-9339
Website: http:// www.brain.nwu.edu

Alzheimer's Disease Center
Rush-Presbyterian-St. Luke's Medical Center
Rush Institute for Healthy Aging
1645 West Jackson Boulevard, Suite 675
Chicago IL 60612
Director: Denis Evans, M.D.
Director's telephone: 312-942-3350
Information: 312-942-4463
Website: http:// www.rush.edu/patients/radc/

## Indiana

Indiana Alzheimer's Disease Center
Indiana University School of Medicine
Department of Pathology and Laboratory Medicine
635 Barnhill Drive, MS-A142
Indianapolis, IN 46202-5120
Director: Bernardino Ghetti, M.D.
Information: 317-278-2030
Website: http://www.pathology.iupui.edu/ad/

## Kentucky

Sanders-Brown Research Center on Aging
University of Kentucky
101 Sanders-Brown Building
Lexington KY 40536-0230
Director: William Markesbery, M.D.
Director's telephone: 606-323-6040
Website: http://www.coa.uky.edu/

## Maryland

Alzheimer's Disease Center
Division of Neuropathology
The Johns Hopkins University School of Medicine
558 Ross Research Building
720 Rutland Avenue
Baltimore, MD 21205-2196
Director: Donald Price, M.D.
Director's telephone: 410-955-5632

## Massachusetts

Alzheimer's Disease Center
GRECC Program (182B)
Bedford VAMC
200 Springs Road
Bedford MA 01730
Director: Neil William Kowall, M.D.
Director's telephone: 781-687-2632
Information: 781-687-2916
Website: http://www.xfaux.com/Alzheimer/

Alzheimer's Disease Center
Department of Neurology
Massachusetts General Hospital
15 Parkman Street
Boston MA 02114
Director: John Growdon, M.D.
Director's telephone: 617-726-1728

## Michigan

University of Michigan
Department of Neurology
1500 E. Medical Center Drive
1914 Taubman Street
Ann Arbor, MI 48109-0316
Director: Sid Gilman, M.D.
Director's telephone: 734-936-9070
Information: 734-764-2190
Website: http://www.med.umich.edu/madrc/

## Minnesota

Department of Neurology
Mayo Clinic
200 First Street SW
Rochester MN 55905
Director: Ronald Petersen, M.D.
Director's telephone: 507-538-0487
Information: 507-284-1324
Website: http:// www.mayo.edu/research/alzheimers_center/

## Missouri

Alzheimer's Disease Research Center
Washington University Medical Center
4488 Forest Park Avenue
St. Louis, MO 63108-2293
Directors: Eugene Johnson Jr., Ph.D. & John Morris, M.D.
Director's telephone: 314-286-2881
Information: 314-286-2881
Website: http://www.biostat.wustl.edu/adrc/

## New York

Alzheimer's Disease Center
Columbia University
Department of Pathology
630 West 168th Street
New York NY 10032
Director: Michael Shelanski, M.D., Ph.D.
Director's telephone: 212-305-3300
Information: 212-305-6553
Website: http://pathology.cpmc.columbia.edu/adhome.html/

Department of Psychiatry, Box 1230
Mount Sinai School of Medicine
One Gustave L. Levy Place
New York NY 10029-6574
Director: Kenneth Davis, M.D.
Director's telephone: 212-824-7008
Information: 212-241-8329
Website: http:// www.mssm.edu/psychiatry/adrchome.html/

Alzheimer's Disease Center
New York University School of Medicine
550 First Avenue Room THN 312B
New York NY 10016
Director: Steven Ferris, Ph.D.
Director's telephone: 212-263-5703
Information: 212-263-5700
Website: http://aging.med.nyu.edu/

Alzheimer's Disease Center
Center for Aging and Developmental Biology
University of Rochester Medical Center
601 Elmwood Avenue Box 645
Rochester NY 14642
Director: Paul Coleman, Ph.D.
Director's telephone: 716-275-2581
Information: 716-275-2581
Website: http:// www.urmc.rochester.edu/adc/index.html/

## North Carolina

Joseph and Kathleen Bryan Alzheimer's Disease Research Center
2200 West Main Street, Suite A-230
Durham NC 27705
Director: Donald Schmechel, M.D.
Director's telephone: 919-286-3228
Information: 919-286-3228
Website: http:// www.medicine.mc.duke.edu/adrc/

## Ohio

University Alzheimer Center
University Hospitals of Cleveland
Case Western Reserve University
12220 Fairhill Road
Cleveland, OH 44120-1013
Director: Karl Herrup, Ph.D.
Director's telephone: 216-844-6422
Information: 800-252-5048
Website: http:// www.ohioalzcenter.org/

## Oregon

Alzheimer's Disease Center
Department of Neurology, CR 131
Oregon Health Sciences University
3181 SW Sam Jackson Park Road
Portland, OR 97201-3098
Director: Jeffrey Kaye, M.D.
Director's telephone: 503-494-6976
Information: 503-494-6976
Website: http:// www.ohsu.edu/som-alzheimers/

## Pennsylvania

Alzheimer's Disease Center
Center for Neurodegenerative Disease Research
University of Pennsylvania School of Medicine
3rd Floor Maloney Building
3600 Spruce Street
Philadelphia PA 19104-4283
Director: John Trojanowski, M.D., Ph.D.
Director's telephone: 215-662-6399
Information: 215-662-4708
Website: http:// www.med.upenn.edu/cndr/

Alzheimer's Disease Center
University of Pittsburgh
4-West Montefiore University Hospital
200 Lothrop Street
Pittsburgh, PA 15213
Director: Steven DeKosky, M.D.
Director's telephone: 412-624-6889
Information: 412-692-2700
Website: http://www.adrc.pitt.edu/

## Texas

Alzheimer's Disease Center
Department of Neurology
Baylor College of Medicine
6501 Fannin Street NB302
Houston, TX 77030-3498
Director: Stanley Appel, M.D.
Director's telephone: 713-798-4073
Information: 713-798-6660
Website: http:// www.bcm.tmc.edu/neurol/struct/adrc/adrc1.html

Alzheimer's Disease Research Center
University of Texas Southwestern Medical Center
Southwestern Medical Center
5323 Harry Hines Boulevard
Dallas, TX 75235-9036
Director: Roger Rosenberg, M.D.
Director's telephone: 214-648-3239
Information: 214-648-3198
Website: http:// www.swmed.edu/home_pages/alzheimer

## Washington

Alzheimer's Disease Center
Department of Psychiatry
VA Medical Center
GRECC (116A)
1660 S. Columbian Way
Seattle WA 98108
Director: Murray Raskind, M.D.
Director's telephone: 206-768-5304
Information: 206-277-3491
Website: http://www.depts.washington.edu/adrcweb/

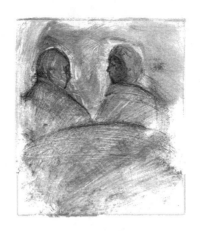

# Appendix B

# Resources For Caregivers

The resources listed in this Appendix offer valuable information on many aspects of Alzheimer's disease. The names, web addresses, and contact information are included for each organization or website. For easy reference, the list is in alphabetical order under each subject. If you are not familiar with Internet use, a quick guide and helpful tips follows this list. If you do not have Internet access, contact your local library for information about free computer instructions and Internet use.

We have included a very important section on evaluating health-related websites following this list. Please read it carefully. *A NOTE OF CAUTION: Although many valuable websites exist on the Internet, some are not as reliable for accuracy as others. Although we can never be certain about the accuracy of information on any website, we believe these to be reliable. Mention of any website addresses in this Appendix does not imply endorsement by the authors or publisher of this book.*

A few sites listed below include tips on finding Alzheimer's information, but websites occasionally change their home page design. In most cases, typing in "Alzheimer's disease" in the search box will take you to the right location.

# Information on Many Aspects
## of Alzheimer's

**American Association of Retired People (AARP)** - www.aarp.org
601 E St. NW, Washington, DC 20049 – Phone: 800-424-3410
This site includes valuable information about caregiving, legal issues, community services, home health care, nursing home issues.

**Alzheimer's Association** - www.alz.org
919 N. Michigan Ave., Suite 1100, Chicago, IL 60611 – Phone: 800-272-3900
The site offers a wealth of information about Alzheimer's disease and resources for caregivers.

**American Medical Association** - www.ama-assn.org
515 N. State St., Chicago, IL 60610 – Phone: 312-464-5000
Information on many diseases, including Alzheimer's information. You will also find other site links for Alzheimer's. Some articles in Spanish.

**Administration on Aging (AOA)** - www.aoa.dhhs.gov
330 Independence Ave., SW, Washington, DC 20201.
Phone for Eldercare Locator (To find services for an older person in his or her locality) 800-677-1116 (Also available in Spanish)
Click on site index for caregiving and Alzheimer-related issues.
• You also can call the National Institute of Aging toll-free at 1-800-438-4380

**Alzheimer Solutions** - www.caregiving-solutions.com
3122 Knorr St., Philadelphia, PA 19149 – Phone: 215-624-2098
*NOTE: This website is owned and maintained by Jim Knittweis.* Features the latest in medical research news on Alzheimer's disease, including information about Alzheimer drugs. You'll find evaluation tests and caregiving links to many other Alzheimer-related websites. A line of products for caregivers and their patients is offered.

**Healthfinder** - www.healthfinder.gov
A searchable list of many health-related information sources from the U.S. government.

**National Institutes of Health** - www.NIH.gov
Bethesda, MD 20892 – Information Hotline For Alzheimer's: 800-438-4380.
Offers information on a wide variety of topics. But very specific information about Alzheimer's disease can be found on this site by clicking on NIH Health Information Index. Also find Alzheimer's Disease Education & Referral (ADEAR), which lists many publications, including caregiving books.

**New York Online Access to Health** - www.noah-health.org/index
A full-text, user-friendly health information site for consumers.
Entire site is offered in English and Spanish.

# Medicine and Research

**Dementia Web** – www.dementia.ion.ucl.ac.uk
Site of a research group supported by the Institute of Neurology and the Division of Neurosciences, Imperial College School of Medicine in London. You will find subjects such as Counseling & Diagnosis in Dementia, Quality Research, Young Onset Dementia, and Dementia Drug Guidelines. It also offers a Virtual Carer Support Chat Room.

**John Douglas French Alzheimer's Foundation** - www.jdfaf.org
11620 Wilshire Blvd., Suite 270, Los Angeles, CA 90025.
A nonprofit public charity funding new research frontiers. Tells how to obtain a free information pamphlet about caregiving and research updates by contacting the foundation by e-mail.

**Mayo Clinic** - www.mayoclinic.com
200 First St., SW, Rochester, MN 55905 – Phone: 507-284-2433
For a list of discussions and research regarding Alzheimer's, use the box marked "For." Type the words "Alzheimer's disease." To receive more general information about Alzheimer's, click on "Diseases & Conditions," then click on "Alzheimer's disease."

**National Center for Complementary and Alternative Medicine (NCCAM) at the National Institutes of Health (NIH)** - www.nccam.gov
NCCAM Clearinghouse, P.O.Box 8218, Silver Spring, MD 20907 – Phone: 888-644-6226.
Site offers information about complementary and alternative medicine. It also offers cautionary information about alternative medicines. You can contact NCCAM toll free at 1-888-644-6226.

**Pharmaceutical Research and Manufacturers of America** - www.phrma.org
1100 Fifteenth St., NW, Washington, DC 20005 – Phone: 202-835-3400
This website lists member pharmaceutical companies that offer free medications through physicians to patients who could not otherwise afford them.

- In the search box, type "free medications for senior citizens."

**Doctor's Guide to the Internet** - www.pslgroup.com/ALZHEIMER.htm
Contains the latest medical news and information on Alzheimer research. Updates discuss new drugs available for treating Alzheimer's disease.

# *Caregiving Educational Information*

**Washington University in St. Louis** - www.biostat.wustl.edu/alzheimer/ The Alzheimer's page is called "The Internet Gateway for the Alzheimer's List," which is a free e-mail based support group for family caregivers and professionals. It features an online chat group where caregivers can send messages to each other.

**Empowering Caregivers** - www.care-givers.com Inspirational and spiritual in tone. Offers a newsletter, useful caregiving tips, and a message board for caregivers to talk about their problems with one another.

- Go to this homepage and click on "Enter Caregivers.com."

- For message board, click on "Forums – Message Boards". First-time users instructions are offered.

**Today's Caregiver Magazine** - www.caregiver.com
6365 Taft St., Suite #3006, Hollywood, FL 33024 – Phone: 954-893-0550.
Website for the first national magazine dedicated to caregivers. The website includes topic-specific newsletters, online discussion lists, back issue articles from the magazine, and chat room.

**American Dietetic Association** - www.eatright.org
216 W. Jackson Blvd., Chicago, IL 60606 – Phone: 312-899-0040 (Also in Spanish)
Offers a great deal of information about nutrition and health.

**U. S. Food & Drug Administration** - www.fda.gov
5600 Fishers Lane, Rockville, MD 20857 – Phone: For Information and to order publications – 888-463-6332
Information about Alzheimer-related and other FDA publications are available online or as reprints (selected publications are also in Spanish).

- Click on site map. Click on publications.

134

# Care Facilities and Agencies and Housing Options

**American Association of Homes and Services for the Aging** - www.aahsa.org
2519 Connecticut Ave., NW, Washington, DC 20008 – 202-783-2242. This nonprofit organization represents nursing homes, assisted-living facilities, and community agencies. Website offers information for consumers and family caregivers.

**American Health Care Association** - www.ahca.org Phone: 800-628-8140
A federation of organizations representing long-term care providers. Offers a consumer's guide to nursing facilities and assisted living information. Provides addresses for all state affiliates of the association on website.

**Assisted Living Federation of America** - www.alfa.org
11200 Waples Mill Rd., Suite 150, Fairfax, VA 22030 – Phone: 703-691-8100.
A nonprofit organization that offers information on assisted-living facilities throughout the U.S.

- Go to Homepage and click on "Consumers."

**Hospice Net** - www.hospicenet.org
Suite 51, 401 Bowling Ave., Nashville, TN 37205
Offers information on hospice care for caregivers wanting to place an advanced dementia patient in a hospice.

**Medicare Nursing Home Comparisons** – www.medicare.gov/NHCompare/home.asp Takes you directly to U.S. Government comparison of nursing homes in the U.S. For Medicare and Social Security Benefits information – Phone: 800-772-1213

**The National Council on Aging** - www.ncoa.org
409 Third St., SW, Suite 200, Washington, DC 20024 – Phone: 202-479-1200.
Information on Adult Day Care Services – locating them and rating them. Information includes "Choosing a Center," which offers information on how to select an adult day services center and how to locate an adult day care center near you.

- Go to this homepage. Click on "Visitors Center"

- On left side see "Constituent Units" – click on it

- Click on "NADSA (National Adult Day Services Association)

**Visiting Nurse Associations of America (VNAA)** – www.vnaa.org
11 Beacon St., Suite 910, Boston, MA 02108 – Phone: 617-523-4042. The VNAA is the national association of freestanding not-for-profit, community-based visiting nurse agencies. Learn how to choose and locate a local visiting nurse agency and what types of home healthcare services and personnel are available. Also answers commonly asked questions about home care including how to pay for services.

# Legal Information

**National Senior Citizens Law Center** - www.nsclc.org
1101 14<sup>th</sup> St., NW, Suite 400, Washington, DC 20005 – Phone: 202-289-6976.
Nonprofit group that advocates for legal rights for older individuals with disabilities and for low income elderly.

- Go to this homepage, click on Consumer's page for legal issues.

**National Academy of Elder Law Attorneys** – www.naela.com
1604 N. Country Club Rd., Tucson, AZ 85716 – Phone: 520-881-4005
Elder law resources, publications available list, questions to ask when choosing an attorney.

# Family Support Information

**National Family Caregivers Association** - www.nfcacares.org
10400 Connecticut Ave., #500, Kensington, MD 20895 – Phone: 800-896-3650.
An organization created to support, educate, and empower Americans who care for chronically ill, aged, or disabled loved ones. The organization offers free membership to family caregivers. To become a member:

- Go to homepage, click on "Join NFCA." No fee is charged for membership. It also offers many free or low-cost publications such as "Faith Community Outreach Kit," and "NFCA's Bereavement Kits" among others. To find the list of publications:

- Go to homepage, click on "Services".

*The following are websites from the above list that include chat rooms and message boards for Alzheimer caregivers:*
www.biostat.wustl.edu/alzheimer/
www.care-givers.com
www.caregiver.com
www.dementia.ion.ucl.ac.uk

# Evaluating Health-related Websites

*Be very careful to check the validity of the information found on all Internet websites, and especially health-related information. The following websites will help evaluate their content.*

**The Highlands Regional Library Cooperative -** www.hrlc.org/healthsavvy.htm
An excellent and objective web address for evaluating health-related Internet websites. The information was gathered by the Highlands Regional Library Cooperative in New Jersey with a grant from the National Network of Libraries of Medicine.

- Go to web address. Click on "Evaluating Health Websites"

**Senior Net Health Site Evaluation -** www.seniornet.org/healtheval
Direct link to the seniornet.org health site evaluation. (You will see more information about this site below. See "A Good Place to Start.")

**Gomez -** www.gomez.com The website evaluates its top ten choices for best websites for a multitude of categories. Health-related websites are included. Gomez tells you why and how they chose those particular websites.

# Information for First-time Internet Users

*Tips to Remember – Internet Web Addresses*

- Whenever a period (.) or a hyphen (-) appears in a web address, be sure to include it in exactly the correct spot.

- When typing a web address that includes a slash, make sure to use the correct slash mark. The one on the question (?) key is known as a front slash. The other slash on the keyboard is known as a back slash.

- Some web addresses end in .htm and some end in .html – use the correct one. The websites offered in this Appendix are easy to use if you follow the following steps.

# Step-by-Step Guide For Using These Websites

- In the address box, carefully type in the listed address.

- Always use the left click on your mouse to navigate pages.

- When the web page appears, you will likely find a box named "Search," or "Find." With most sites, typing the words "Alzheimer's disease" will bring you the information you want. Once you type in your topic, click on the "Go" or "Search" box or push the Enter key on your keyboard.

- As each new page comes up, read it over to see what information your want or where you want to go next. (Most websites offer a "Help" button for searches.)

- As you move from page to page, continue to click on the topic you want. If you should reach a page, then decide it does not give the information you want, go to your toolbar and click on "Back." That will take you to the preceding page so that you may make a new choice without leaving the website. If you accidentally lose the website, just simply enter the web address and start over.

- Many of the websites listed in this appendix offer links to other sites. You can reach these links simply by clicking on the www. address to the links. Remember: when you go to a link, you may have disconnected from the original website. If you want to return to it, just retype the website address in the address box.

# A Good Place to Get Started

**Senior Net -** www.seniornet.com
121 Second St., 7<sup>th</sup> Floor, San Francisco, CA 94105 – Phone: 415-495-4990
This nonprofit website offers a free tutorial for beginners on how to use the Internet. Look on the home page for "Free Searching the Internet Course." It is a self-paced, four-lesson tutorial. (The website offers information relevant to those 50 years and older, but anyone can use the site, regardless of age). A glossary is included.

# *Also Available On This Website:*

- A SeniorNet Roundtable Discussion. This discussion is free. You do not have to join SeniorNet to partake in the roundtable discussions. The discussions allow people to chat with one another along with a professional to guide them.

- An excellent feature for Alzheimer caregivers is the "Health Site Evaluation." As always, it is important to know the credibility of the source of information you receive from the Internet.

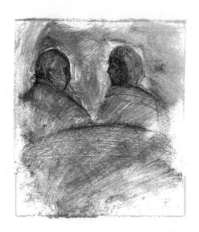

# *Appendix C*

# *Choosing A Nursing Home*

The best time to begin searching for a good nursing home is when your loved one is first diagnosed with Alzheimer's. Most nursing homes have long waiting lists. Caregivers frequently discover that it is almost impossible to find a nursing home quickly.

Inevitably, the disease process will bring many caregivers to the realization that their patient needs round-the-clock care. Once the decision is made to place your loved one in a nursing home, the challenge of finding one that meets your standards of care and your patient's financial resources can be difficult and time-consuming. By doing your research early, you will have a good head start.

*What types of nursing homes are there?*

- Public nursing homes – owned by state/local governments

- Voluntary nursing homes – not-for-profit businesses

- Proprietary nursing homes – businesses operated for profit

140

*Are there any organizations to help in my search?*

- Volunteer groups working with the elderly and chronically ill. (See Appendix B)

- Clergy and religious organizations can help you find a religion-based nursing home for your patient. Check with the leaders of your house of worship.

- The Long-Term Care Ombudsman Program operates through your state's office of aging. There are more than 800 state and local ombudsmen in the U.S. Their mission is to protect the health, safety, welfare and rights of the elderly.

- To find the ombudsman in your state, call your state office of aging or visit www.angelfire.com/tn/NursingHome/index.html. Click on directory of "Ombudsman for All States."

Beginning research early will allow you to look at many options in the selection process. Your search will be easier if you consult a social worker knowledgeable in nursing home placement.

*How can I find a professional to help me locate a nursing home?*

- Contact your local or county Office of Aging. Virtually every county in the U.S. has a local area agency on aging. They can assist you in finding a social worker.

- To find a licensed social worker with strong educational credentials, contact the National Association of Social Workers. Address: 750 First St., NE, Suite 700, Washington, DC 20002 Telephone number: toll-free at 800-638-8799 or 202-408-8600. Web address: www.naswdc.org - Website offers the Register of Clinical Social Workers. Conduct an online search to find a clinical social worker by state or zip code at www.naswdc.org/register/disclaimer.htm. Click on "I accept and would like to begin my search." When the search box appears, fill in boxes for zip code, city, and state. Under "Client Group," select "geriatric." You will find a list of clinical social workers that specialize in working with the elderly.

- If your patient is being treated at a major Alzheimer's Disease Center (see Appendix A for a state-by-state listing), ask the center director for the name of the resident social worker. The social worker will talk with you to determine your preferences in nursing homes and will supply you with details about nursing homes in your area. In many cases, social workers, in conjunction with your patient's physician, can help make arrangements for admittance to a nursing home.

*Are there any other health professionals I can turn to for nursing home advice?*

Yes. Another excellent source of professional help is the National Association of Geriatric Care Managers. A geriatric care manager is a professional who specializes in assisting older people and their families in meeting their long-term care arrangements, including selection of a nursing home. Some geriatric care managers also provide assistance with financial and legal issues.

*How can I find a geriatric care manager?*

- Contact the National Association of Geriatric Care Managers at 1604 N. Country Club Road, Tucson, Arizona 85716. Telephone number: 520-881-8008.

- Go to the association's web page address: www.caremanager.org/gcm/ProfCareManagers1.htm, click on "How to Find A Care Manager." Then search by state or zip code to find a geriatric care manager in your area.

*Who else can I consult about nursing home choices?*

*Note: When you receive advice about nursing homes, remember to ask if those nursing homes have the proper facilities and staff for Alzheimer patients.*

- If your patient is being moved from a hospital, talk with the discharge staff. They will help you find an appropriate nursing home for your patient's specific needs.

- Call your local government health department for information.

- Ask family and friends about their own experiences with nursing homes.

- If you know someone living in a nursing home, visit that person and ask questions about the facility.

- Ask members of volunteer community or religious organizations. They may be knowledgeable about the quality of area nursing homes through member feedback.

*What other resources are available for nursing home information?*

- See Appendix B – *Resources for Caregivers.* Under "Care Facilities and Agencies and Housing Options," you will find contact information for:

  - The American Association of Homes and Services for the Aging

  - American Health Care Association

  - Assisted Living Federation of America

  - Medicare Nursing Home Comparisons

- Other sites listed under *Information on Many Aspects of Alzheimer's* in Appendix B such as the AARP and the Alzheimer's Association offer a great deal of information about nursing home selection on their websites.

- Seniorsite.com (www.seniorsite.com) has extensive information about evaluating nursing homes, legalities, state regulations, insurance coverage, etc.

*Once I've narrowed down my choice, whom should I talk with at the nursing home?*

Any good nursing home will welcome inquiries by caregivers. Visit the nursing home, check out all its facilities, discuss financial issues frankly, and talk extensively with the following staff members:

- Administrators

- Social workers

- Nursing director

- Physicians

*After I've made my decision, what should I do next?*

- Regulations require formal application before you can be placed on a waiting list. As soon as you've made your choice, fill out required forms, and ask to be placed on the waiting list.

- Continue to check the status of your application. Call the nursing home regularly to see where you stand. Call the specific office to which you submitted your application.

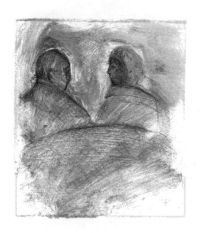

# Appendix D

# Product Resources

**Anti-scalding device for showers**
*Memry Corporation* makes a simple valve that installs on showers and sink faucets without special tools. The valve can be purchased from *TCP Inc.*
Telephone #: 917-817-3389
Website address: www.antiscald.com

**Adult Bibs**
Available from *Alzheimer Solutions*
Telephone #: 215-624-2098
Website address: www.caregiving-solutions.com

**Drinking cups and straws**
Available from *Alzheimer Solutions*
Telephone #: 215-624-2098
Website address: www.caregiving-solutions.com

**Grab Bars**
*Sammons Preston* offers a nice line of affordable grab bars for the bathroom.
Toll-free #: 800-323-5547
Website address: www.sammonspreston.com
*Franklin Brass* makes a custom line of grab bars. Some are quite attractive.
Telephone #: 310-885-3200
Website address: www.franklinbrass.com

***Suction Cup Dish***
This dish has suction cups on the bottom of the plate to keep the plate from being knocked off a table. Available from: www.caregiving-solutions.com

***Swivel spoons***
This spoon swivels and pivots, allowing people with poor hand motion to easily feed themselves. Available from: www.caregiving-solutions.com

***Thick N Easy***
This product is for patients having difficulty swallowing food. When added to food, it gives the food extra consistency so that it can be more easily swallowed. Thick N Easy is made by *Hormel*.
Available from: www.caregiving-solutions.com

***Wandering alarms and devices***
*Care Electronics* makes the WanderCare alarm system, which triggers an alarm when a preset distance is breeched by the patient.
Telephone #: 303-444-2273
Website address: www.careelectronics.com

***Care Trak Inc.*** makes the Care Trak alarm system. This system is used by police departments to locate patients who have wandered as far away as up to one mile from home. The company rents the system to customers.
Toll-free telephone #: 800-842-4537
Website address: www.caretrak.com

***Home Technology Systems*** makes the Data Wave Door Contact. Whenever a patient opens a door, a chime sounds on the receiver, which is kept near the caregiver.
Toll-free telephone #: 800-922-3555.
Website address: www.hometechsystems.com

***Instantel Inc.*** makes the Watch Mate System. When a patient enters a forbidden area such as a pool or a door, a transmitter worn by the patient sets off an alarm. A monitor displays the location of the patient.
Toll-free telephone#: 800-267-9111
Website address: www.instantel.com

# Glossary

When you become a caregiver for an Alzheimer's patient, your world is suddenly filled with new terminology. Health care professionals sometimes speak in medical jargon. These terms are so familiar to them that they may forget to explain the meanings to you.

The following terms and definitions are used with the permission of the Alzheimer's Association. We have excluded much of the scientific terminology that is included on the Alzheimer's Association list, but you can obtain the complete listing at the association's website at www.alz.org (click on the heading "Glossary" on the homepage).

Legal and financial terminology from the Alzheimer's Association's Glossary is listed separately. It follows the glossary below.

# A

**Abilities** – Level at which certain actions and activities can be carried out.

**Activities of daily living (ADLs)** – Personal care activities necessary for everyday living, such as eating, bathing, grooming, dressing, and toileting. People with dementia may not be able to perform necessary functions without assistance. Professionals often assess a person's ADLs to determine what type of care is needed.

**Adult day services** – programs that provide participants with opportunities to interact with others, usually in a community center or facility. Staff lead various activities such as music programs and support groups. Transportation is often provided.

**Adverse reaction** – An unexpected effect of drug treatment that may be serious or life-threatening, such as an allergic reaction.

**Aggression** – Hitting, pushing, or threatening behavior that commonly occurs when a caregiver attempts to help an individual with Alzheimer's with daily activities, such as dressing. It is important to control such behavior because aggressive persons can cause injury to themselves and others.

**Agitation** – Vocal or motor behavior (screaming, shouting, complaining, moaning, cursing, pacing, fidgeting, wandering, etc.) that is disruptive, unsafe, or interferes with the delivery of care in a particular environment. An abnormal behavior is considered agitation only if it poses risk or discomfort to the individual with Alzheimer's or his/her caregiver. Agitation can be a nonspecific symptom of one or more physical or psychological problems (e.g., headache, depression).

**Alzheimer's disease** – A progressive, neurodegenerative disease characterized by loss of function and death of nerve cells in several areas of the brain, leading to loss of mental functions such as memory and learning. Alzheimer's disease is the most common cause of dementia.

**Ambulation** – The ability to walk and move about freely.

**Amyloid** – A protein deposit associated with tissue degeneration; amyloid is found in the brains of individuals with Alzheimer's.

**Amyloid plaque** – Abnormal cluster of dead and dying nerve cells, other brain cells, and amyloid protein fragments. Amyloid plaques are one of the characteristic structural abnormalities found in the brains of individuals with Alzheimer's. Upon autopsy, the presence of amyloid plaques and neurofibrillary tangles is used to positively diagnose Alzheimer's.

**Antibodies** – Specialized proteins produced by the cells of the immune system that counteract a specific foreign substance. The production of antibodies is the first line of defense in the body's immune system.

**Anti-inflammatory drugs** – Drugs that reduce inflammation by modifying the body's immune system.

**Anxiety** – A feeling of apprehension, fear, nervousness, or dread accompanied by restlessness or tension.

**Apathy** – Lack of interest, concern, or emotion.

**Aphasia** – Difficulty understanding others and/or expressing oneself verbally.

**Art therapy** – A form of therapy that allows people with dementia opportunities to express their feelings creatively through art.

**Assessment** – An evaluation, usually performed by a physician, of a person's mental, emotional, and social capabilities.

**Assisted living facility** – A residential care setting that combines housing, support services, and health care for people typically in the early or middle stages of Alzheimer's disease.

**Autonomy** – A person's ability to make independent choices.

# B

**Behavioral symptoms** – In Alzheimer's disease, symptoms that relate to action or emotion, such as wandering, depression, anxiety, hostility, and sleep disturbances.

# C

**Caregiver** – The primary person in charge of caring for an individual with Alzheimer's disease, usually a family member or a designated health care professional.

**Care planning** – A written action plan containing strategies for delivering care that address an individual's specific needs or problems.

**Case management** – A term used to describe formal services planned by care professionals.

**Coexisting illness** – A medical condition that exists simultaneously with another, such as arthritis and dementia.

**Cognitive abilities** – Mental abilities such as judgment, memory, learning, comprehension, and reasoning.

**Cognitive symptoms** – In Alzheimer's disease, the symptoms that relate to loss of thought processes, such as learning, comprehension, memory, reasoning, and judgment.

**Combativeness** – Incidents of aggression.

**Competence** – A person's ability to make informed choices.

**CT scan** (computed tomography) - A type of imaging scan that shows the internal structure of a person's brain. In diagnosing dementia, CT scans reveals tumors and small strokes in the brain.

**Continuum of care** – Care services available to assist individuals throughout the course of the disease.

**Cueing** – The process of providing cues, prompts, hints, and other meaningful information, direction, or instruction to aid a person who is experiencing memory difficulties.

# D

**Deficits** – Physical and/or cognitive skills or abilities that a person has lost, has difficulty with, or can no longer perform due to his or her dementia.

**Delusion** – A false idea typically originating from a misinterpretation but firmly believed and strongly maintained in spite of contradictory proof or evidence.

**Dementia** – The loss of intellectual functions (such as thinking, remembering, and reasoning) of sufficient severity to interfere with a person's daily functioning. Dementia is not a disease itself but rather a group of symptoms that may accompany certain diseases or conditions. Symptoms may also include changes in personality, mood, and behavior. Dementia is irreversible when caused by disease or injury but may be reversible when caused by drugs, alcohol, hormone or vitamin imbalances, or depression.

**Dementia-capable** – Skilled in working with people with dementia and their caregivers, knowledgeable about the kinds of services that may help them, and aware of which agencies and individuals provide such services.

**Dementia-specific** – Services that are provided specifically for people with dementia.

**Disorientation** – A cognitive disability in which the senses of time, direction, and recognition become difficult to distinguish.

# E

**Early-onset Alzheimer's disease** – A rare form of Alzheimer's in which individuals are diagnosed with Alzheimer's before the age of 65. Less than 10% of all Alzheimer patients have early-onset. Early-onset Alzheimer's is associated with mutations in genes located on chromosomes 1, 14, and 21.

**Early stage** – The beginning stages of Alzheimer's disease when an individual experiences very mild to moderate cognitive impairments.

# F

**Familial Alzheimer's disease** – A form of Alzheimer's disease that runs in families.

# G

**Gait** – A person's manner of walking. People in the later stages of Alzheimer's often have "reduced gait," meaning their ability to lift their feet as they walk has diminished.

# H

**Hoarding** – Collecting and putting things away in a guarded manner.

**Hospice** – Philosophy and approach to providing comfort and care at life's end rather than heroic lifesaving measures.

# I

**Immune system** – A system of cells that protect a person from bacteria, viruses, toxins, and other foreign substances that gain access to the body.

**Incontinence** – Loss of bladder and/or bowel control.

**Instrumental activities of daily living** (IADLs) – Secondary level of activities (different from ADLs, such as eating, dressing, and bathing) important to daily living, such as cooking, writing, and driving.

# J, K, L

**Late-onset Alzheimer's disease** – The most common form of Alzheimer's disease, usually occurring after age 65. Late-onset Alzheimer's strikes almost half of all people over the age of 85 and may or may not be hereditary.

**Late-stage** – Designation given when dementia symptoms have progressed to the extent that a person has little capacity for self-care.

**Layering** – Behavior that involves inappropriately changing or layering clothing on top of one another.

# M

**Mini-Mental State Examination** (MMSE) – A standard mental status exam routinely used to measure a person's basic cognitive skills, such as short-term memory, long-term memory, orientation, writing, and language.

**Music therapy** – Use of music to improve physical, psychological, cognitive, and social functioning.

# N

**Neurological disorder** – Disturbance in structure or function of the nervous system resulting from developmental abnormality, disease, injury, or toxin.

**Neurologist** – A physician who diagnoses and treats disorders of the nervous system.

**Neuropathology** – Changes in the brain produced by a disease.

# O

**Onset** – Defines time of life when Alzheimer's disease begins (e.g., early-onset, late-onset).

# P

**Pacing** – Aimless wandering, often triggered by an internal stimulus (e.g., pain, hunger, or boredom) or some distraction in the environment (e.g., noise, smell, temperature).

**Paranoia** – Suspicion of others that is not based on fact.

**Perseveration** – Persistent repetition of an activity, word, phrase, or movement, such as tapping, wiping, and picking.

**Pillaging** – Taking things that belong to someone else. A person with dementia may think something belongs to him/her, even when it clearly does not.

**Placebo** – An inert/innocuous substance – for example, a sugar pill.

# Q

**Quality care** – Term used to describe care and services that allow recipients to attain and maintain their highest level of mental, physical, and psychological function, in a dignified and caring way.

# R

**Reassurance** – Encouragement intended to relieve tension, fear, and confusion that can result from dementing illnesses.

**Reinforcement** –Employment of praise, repetition, and stimulation of the senses to preserve a person's memory, capabilities, and level of self-assurance.

**Reminiscence** – Life review activity aimed at surfacing and reviewing positive memories and experiences.

**Repetitive behaviors** – Repeated questions, stories, and outbursts or specific activities done over and over again, common in people with dementia.

**Respite** – A short break or time away.

**Respite care** – Services that provide people with temporary relief from tasks associated with caregiving (e.g., in-home assistance, short nursing home stays, adult day care).

**Restraints** – Devices used to ensure safety by restricting and controlling a person's movement. Many facilities are "restraint free" or use alternative methods to help modify behavior.

**Risk factors** – Factors that have been shown to increase one's odds of developing a disease. In Alzheimer's disease, the only established risk factors are age, family history, and genetics.

# S

**Safe Return** – The Alzheimer's Association's nationwide identification, support, and registration program that assists in the safe return of individuals with Alzheimer's or related dementia who wander and become lost.

**Senility** – Term meaning "old," once used to describe elderly diagnosed with dementia. Today, we know dementia is caused by various diseases (e.g., Alzheimer's) and is not a normal part of aging.

**Sequencing** – Doing things in a logical, predictable order.

**Shadowing** – Following, mimicking, interrupting behaviors that people with dementia may experience.

**Skilled nursing care** – Level of care that includes ongoing medical or nursing services.

**Special care unit** – Designated area of a residential care facility or nursing home that cares specifically for the needs of people with Alzheimer's.

**Stages** – Course of disease progression defined by levels or periods of severity; early, mild, moderate, moderately severe, severe.

**Sundowning** – Unsettled behavior evident in the late afternoon or early evening.

**Support group** – Facilitated gathering of caregivers, family, friends, or others affected by a disease or condition for the purpose of discussing issues related to the disease.

**Suspiciousness** – A mistrust common in Alzheimer patients as their memory becomes progressively worse. A common example is when patients believe their glasses or other belongings have been stolen because they forgot where they left them.

# T

**Trigger** – An environmental or personal stimulus that sets off particular and sometimes challenging behavior.

# U, V, W

**Wandering** – Common behavior that causes people with dementia to stray and become lost in familiar surroundings.

# X, Y, Z

# Legal and Financial Terms

**Advance directives** – Written documents, completed and signed when a person is legally competent, that explain a person's medical wishes in advance, allowing someone else to make treatment decisions on his or her behalf later in the disease process.

**Agent** – The individual – usually a trusted family member or friend – authorized by a power of attorney to make legal decisions for another individual.

**Beneficiary** – An individual named in a will who is designated to receive all or part of an estate upon the death of a will maker.

**Conservator** – In some states, the guardian who manages an individual's assets.

**Durable Power of Attorney** – A legal document that allows an individual (the principal) an opportunity to authorize an agent (usually a trusted family member or friend) to make legal decisions for when the person is no longer able to do so themselves.

**Durable Power of Attorney for health care** – A legal document that allows an individual to appoint an agent to make all decisions regarding health care, including choices regarding health care providers, medical treatment, and, in the later stages of the disease, end-of-life decisions.

**Elder law attorney** – An attorney who practices in the area of elder law, a specialized area of law focusing on issues that typically affect older adults.

**Guardian** – An individual appointed by the courts who is authorized to make legal and financial decisions for another individual.

**Living trust** – A legal document that allows an individual (the grantor or trustor) to create a trust and appoint someone else as trustee (usually a trusted individual or bank) to carefully invest and manage his or her assets.

**Living will** – A legal document that expresses an individual's decision on the use of artificial life support systems.

**Medicaid** – A program sponsored by the federal government and administered by states that is intended to provide health care and health-related services to low-income individuals.

**Medicare** – A federal health insurance program for people age 65 and older and for individuals with disabilities.

**Principal** – The individual signing the power of attorney to authorize another individual to legally make decisions for him or her.

**Trustee** – The individual or bank managing the assets of the living trust.

**Will** – A legal document created by an individual that names an executor (the person who will manage the estate) and beneficiaries (persons who will receive the estate at the time of death).

# BIBLIOGRAPHY

Alzheimer's Association (2001) 2001 *Public Publications Catalog*, Alzheimer's Disease and Disorders Association, Inc.

Alzheimer's Association (1998) *Alzheimer's Disease: A Guide For Law Enforcement Officials*, Alzheimer's Disease and Related Disorders Association, Inc.

Alzheimer's Association (2001) *Driving & Dementia*, ED 247ZG, Alzheimer's Disease and Related Disorders Association, Inc.

Bergman-Evans, B., et al. (1994) A Health Profile of Spousal Alzheimer's Caregivers. *Journal of Psychosocial Nursing*, 32:25-30.

Bodnar, J., et al. (1994) Caregiver Depression After Bereavement: Chronic Stress Isn't Over When It's Over. *Psychology and Aging*, 9: 372-380.

Borden, W., et al. (1990) Gender, Coping, and Psychological Well-being in Spouses of Older Adults With Chronic Dementia. *American Journal of Orthopsychiatry*, 60: 603-610.

Boss, P., et al. (1990) Predictors of Depression in Caregivers of Dementia Patients: Boundary Ambiguity and Mastery. *Family Process*, 29: 245-254.

Brown, P., et al. (1991) Australian Caregivers of Family Members with Dementia. *Journal of Gerontological Nursing*, 17: 25-29.

Caserta, M., et al. (1987) Caregivers to Dementia Patients: The Utilization of Community Services. *Gerontologist*, 27: 209-214.

Chenowith, B., et al. (1986) Dementia: The Experience of Family Caregivers. *Gerontologist*, 26: 267-272.

Clipp, E., et al. (1990) Psychotropic Drug Use Among Caregivers of Patients With Dementia. *Journal of the American Geriatrics Society*, 38: 227-235.

Cohen, C., et al. (1994) The Role of Caregiver Social Networks in Alzheimer's Disease. *Social Science and Medicine*, 38: 1483-1490.

Conlin, M., et al. (1992) Reduction of Caregiver Stress by Respite Care. *Southern Medical Journal*, 85: 1096-1100.

Corcoran, M., (1992) Gender Differences in Dementia Management Plans of Spousal Caregivers: Implications for Occupational Therapy. *The American Journal of Occupational Therapy*, 46: 1006-1012.

Cox, C., (1995) Comparing the Experiences of Black and White Caregivers of Dementia Patients. *Social Work*, 40: 343-349.

Cox, C., et al. (1993) Hispanic Culture and Family Care of Alzheimer's Patients. *Health and Social Work,* 18: 92-100.

Cox, C., et al. (1996) Strain Among Caregivers: Comparing the Experiences of African American and Hispanic Caregivers of Alzheimer's Relatives. *International Journal of Aging and Human Development,* 43: 93-105.

Davies, H., et al. (1992) 'Til Death Do Us Part: Intimacy and Sexuality in the Marriages of Alzheimer's Patients. *Journal of Psychosocial Nursing,* 30: 5- 10.

Dura, J., et al. (1990) Chronic Stress and Depressive Disorders in Older Adults. *Journal of Abnormal Psychology,* 99: 284-290.

Dura, J., et al. (1991) Anxiety and Depressive Disorders in Adult Children Caring for Demented Patients. *Psychology and Aging,* 6: 467-473.

Eastley, R., et al. (1997) Prevalence and Correlates of Aggressive Behaviors Occurring in Patients With Alzheimer's Disease. *International Journal of Geriatric Psychiatry,* 12: 484-487.

Fisher, L., et al. (1994) Alzheimer's Disease: The Impact of the Family on Spouses, Offspring, and In-laws. *Family Process,* 33: 305-325.

Fitting, M., et al. (1986) Caregivers for Dementia Patients: A Comparison of Husbands and Wives. *Gerontologist,* 26: 248-253.

Frenchman, I., et al. (1997) Clinical Experience With Risperidone, Haloperidol, and Thioridazine for Dementia-Associated Behavioral Disturbances. *International Psychogeriatrics,* 9: 431-435.

Fritz, C., et al. (1996) Companion Animals and the Psychological Health of Alzheimer Patients' Caregivers. *Psychological Reports,* 78: 467-481.

Gallagher, D., et al, (1989) Prevalence of Depression in Family Caregivers. *Gerontologist,* 29: 449-456.

George, L., et al. (1986) Caregiver Well-Being: A Multidimensional Examination of Family Caregivers of Demented Adults. *Gerontologist,* 26: 253-259.

Gignac, M., et al. (1996) Caregivers' Appraisals of Efficacy in Coping With Dementia. *Psychology and Aging,* 11: 214-225.

Gonyea, J. (1989) Alzheimer's Disease Support Groups: An Analysis of Their Structure, Format, and Perceived Benefits. *Social Work in Health Care,* 14: 61-72.

Goodman, C., et al. (1990) A Model Telephone Information and Support Program for Caregivers of Alzheimer's Patients. *Gerontologist,* 30: 399-404.

Gwyther, L., (1998) Social Issues of the Alzheimer's Patient and Family, *American Journal of Medicine*, 104: 17S-21S.

Haley, W., et al. (1987) Psychological, Social, and Health Consequences of Caring for a Relative With Senile Dementia. *Journal of the American Geriatrics Society*, 35: 405-411.

Haley, W., et al. (1995) Psychological, Social, and Health Impact of Caregiving: A Comparison of Black and White Dementia Family Caregivers and Noncaregivers. *Psychology and Aging*, 10: 540-552.

Haley, W., et al. (1996) Appraisal, Coping, and Social Support as Mediators of Well-being in Black and White Family Caregivers of Patients With Alzheimer's Disease. *Journal of Consulting and Clinical Psychology*, 64: 121-129.

Hamel, M., et al. (1990) Predictors and Consequences of Aggressive Behavior by Community-Based Dementia Patients. *Gerontologist*, 30: 206-211.

Harris, P., (1993) The Misunderstood Caregiver? A Qualitative Study of the Male Caregiver of Alzheimer's Disease Victims. *Gerontologist*, 33: 551-556.

Irwin M., et al. (1987) Life Events, Depressive Symptoms, and Immune Function. *American Journal of Psychiatry*, 144: 437-441.

Jones, D., et al. (1992) The Experience of Bereavement in Caregivers of Family Members With Alzheimer's Disease. *Image: Journal of Nursing Scholarship*, 24: 172-176.

Kaye, L., et al. (1990) Men as Elder Caregivers: A Response to Changing Families. *American Journal of Orthopsychiatry*, 60: 86-95.

Kiecolt-Glaser, J., et al. (1991) Spousal Caregivers of Dementia Victims: Longitudinal Changes in Immunity and Health. *Psychosomatic Medicine*, 53: 345-362.

Kiecolt-Glaser, J., et al. (1996) Chronic Stress Alters the Immune Response to Influenza Virus Vaccine in Older Adults. *Proceedings of the National Academy of Sciences*, 93: 3043-3047.

Kinney, J., et al. (1989) Hassles and Uplifts of Giving Care to a Family Member with Dementia. *Psychology of Aging*, 4: 402-408.

Larkin, J., et al. (1993) In-Hospital Respite as a Moderator of Caregiver Stress. *Health in Social Work*, 18: 132-138.

Lieberman, M., et al. (1999) The Effects of Family Conflict Resolution and Decision Making on the Provision of Help for an Elder With Alzheimer's Disease. *Gerontologist*, 39: 159-165.

Malonebeach, E., et al. (1991) Current Research Issues in Caregiving to the Elderly. *International Journal of Aging and Human Development*, 32: 103-114.

McCabe, B., et al. (1995) Availability and Utilization of Services. *Journal of Gerontological Nursing,* 21: 14-22.

McCann, J., et al. (1997) Why Alzheimer's Disease is a Women's Health Issue. *Journal of the American Women's Medical Association,* 52: 132-137.

Miller, B., et al. (1992) Gender Differences in Caregiving: Fact or Artifact? *Gerontologist,* 32: 496-507.

Miller, B., et al. (1995) Dietary Changes, Compulsions, and Sexual Behavior in Frontotemporal Degeneration. *Dementia,* 6: 195-199.

Mittelman, M., et al. (1993) An Intervention That Delays Institutionalization of Alzheimer's Disease Patients: Treatment of Spouse-Caregivers. *Gerontologist,* 33: 730-740.

Monahan, D., et al. (1997) Caregiving and Social Support in Two Illness Groups. *Social Work,* 42: 278-287.

Motenko, A., et al. (1989) The Frustrations, Gratifications, and Well-Being of Dementia Caregivers. *Gerontologist,* 29: 166-172.

Mullan, J., (1992) The Bereaved Caregiver: A Prospective Study of Changes in Well-Being. *Gerontologist,* 32: 673-683.

National Center for Health Statistics: Disability Days: United States, (1980) Series 10. Number 143. *NCHS,* 1986.

Neundorfer, M., et al. (1991) Coping and Health Outcomes in Spouse Caregivers of Persons With Dementia. *Nursing Research* 40: 260-265.

Ory, M., et al. (1999) Prevalence and Impact of Caregiving: A Detailed Comparison Between Dementia and Nondementia Caregivers. *Gerontologist,* 39: 177-185.

Paveza, G., et al. (1992) Severe Family Violence and Alzheimer's Disease: Prevalence and Risk Factors. *Gerontologist,* 32: 493-497.

Pearlin, L., et al. (1990) Caregiving and the Stress Process: An Overview of Concepts and Their Measures. *Gerontologist,* 30: 583-594.

Pillemer, K., et al. (1992) Violence and Violent Feelings: What Causes Them Among Family Caregivers? *Journal of Gerontology,* Social Sciences, 47: S165-S172.

Pruchno, R., et al. (1989) Aberrant Behaviors and Alzheimer's Disease: Mental Health Effects on Spouse Caregivers. *Journal of Gerontology,* 44: S177- S182.

Pruchno, R., et al. (1989) Caregiving Spouses: Physical and Mental Health in Perspective. *Journal of the American Geriatrics Society,* 37: 697-705.

Pruchno, R., et al. (1989) Husbands and Wives as Caregivers: Antecedents of Depression and Burden. *Gerontologist,* 29: 159-165.

Rabins, P., et al. (1982) The Impact of Dementia on the Family, *Journal of the American Medical Association,* 248: 333-335.

Russo, J., et al. (1995) Psychiatric Disorders in Spouse Caregivers of Care Recipients With Alzheimer's Disease and Matched Controls: A Diathesis-Stress Model of Psychopathology. *Journal of Abnormal Psychology,* 104: 197-204.

Schulz, R., et al. (1990) Psychiatric and Physical Morbidity Effects of Caregiving. *Journal of Gerontology,* 45: P181-P191.

Schulz, R., et al. (1991) A 2 Year Longitudinal Study of Depression Among Alzheimer's Caregivers. *Psychology and Aging,* 6: 569-578.

Scott, J., et al. (1986) Families of Alzheimer's Victims: Family Support to the Caregivers. *Journal of the American Geriatrics Society,* 34: 348-354.

Semple, S., (1992) Conflict in Alzheimer's Caregiving Families: Its Dimensions and Consequences. *Gerontologist,* 32: 648-655.

Shaw, W., et al. (1997) Longitudinal Analysis of Multiple Indicators of Health Decline Among Spousal Caregivers. *Annals of Behavioral Medicine,* 19: 101-109.

Skaff, M., et al. (1992) Caregiving: Role Engulfment and the Loss of Self. *Gerontologist,* 32: 656-664.

Stephens, M., et al. (1991) Stressors and Well-Being Among Caregivers to Older Adults With Dementia: The In-Home Versus Nursing Home Experience. *Gerontologist,* 31: 217- 223.

Takahashi, M., et al. (1996) Case Report of Sodium Valproate Treatment of Aggression Associated With Alzheimer's Disease. *No To Shinkei,* 48: 757-760.

Toseland, R., et al. (1989) Group Interventions to Support Family Caregivers: A Review and Analysis. *Gerontologist,* 29: 438-448.

Tsai, S., et al. (1999) Inappropriate Sexual Behaviors in Dementia: A Preliminary Report. *Alzheimer Disease and Associated Disorders,* 13: 60-62.

U.S. Congress, Office of Technology Assessment: Technology and Aging in America. Publication Number OTA-BA-264. Washington, D.C. US Government Printing Office June 1985).

Uchino, B., et al. (1994) Construals of Pre-illness Relationship Quality Predict Cardiovascular Response in Family Caregivers of Alzheimer's Disease Victims. *Psychology and Aging,* 9: 113-120.

Visiting Nurse Associations of America (1998) *Caregiver's Handbook, A Complete Guide to Home Health Care,* DK Publishing, Inc.

Vitaliano, P., et al. (1991) Predictors of Burden in Spouse Caregivers of Individuals With Alzheimer's Disease. *Psychology and Aging,* 6: 392-402.

Vitaliano, P., et al. (1996) Weight Changes in Caregivers of Alzheimer's Care Recipients: Psychobehavioral Predictors. *Psychology and Aging,* 11: 155-163.

Williamson, G., et al. (1990) Relationship Orientation, Quality of Prior Relationship, and Distress Among Caregivers of Alzheimer Patients. *Psychology and Aging,* 5: 502-509.

Wright, K., et al. (1991) The Impact of Alzheimer's Disease on the Marital Relationship. *Gerontologist,* 31: 224-237.

Wuest, J., et al. (1994) Becoming Strangers: The Changing Family Caregiving Relationship in Alzheimer's Disease. *Journal of Advanced Nursing,* 20: 437-443.

Yankelovitch, Skelly and White, Inc., (1986) Caregivers of Patients With Dementia: Contract Report prepared for the Office of Technology Assessment, U.S. Congress.

Zeiss, A., et al. (1996) An Observational Study of Sexual Behavior in Demented Male Patients. *Journal of Gerontology A:* Biological Science and Medical Science, 51: M325-M329.

# INDEX

# INDEX

# INDEX

## F

Falls 13,25,36,40,42,48,51-52,102

Familiarity 41

Family conflict 67

Fatigue 63

Fiber 25

Financial issues 68-70

Finger foods 3

Fleet's enema 26

Food

  consistency 2

  dangers 4-5

  taste 7

  temperature 4

## G

Grab bars 16,48

Grief 117-120

Guilt 118-119

## H

Hair care 14

Hallucinations 113

Haloperidol 40

Hearing 34

Heimlich maneuver 2,4,9-10

Hip pads 51

Hoarding 6

Hypertension 83

## I

Immobility 16,30-31

Incontinence 28-29

Insulin 83-84

## L

Legal issues 69-70

## M

Mattress cover 29

Medicaid 69

Medicare 69

Medication 24

Memory box 58

Motion detector 42

Music 2,39

# INDEX

## N

Nail care 15

National Academy of Elder Law Attorneys 69

National Association of Geriatric Care Managers 14

National Association of Social Workers 141

National Family Caregivers Association 67

National Senior Citizens Law Center 69

Nightlights 16,18,52,61

Nursing home placement 109,113,118-119,140-143

## O

Oral hygiene 13

## P

Pain 4,18,36

Paranoia 36,38-39,112,114

Passive motion 30

Pets 101

Pharmaceutical Research and Manufacturers of America 69

Polypharmacy 20

Privacy 13,16,28

## R

Religion 77,100

Respite 96-98

Restlessness 2,17

Restraints 115

Risperidone 40

Ross, Elizabeth Kubler 117

Routine 6,61

## S

Safe Return program 41,43-44

Saliva flow 24

Scopolamine 40

Sensory overload 36

Sexual intimacy 110-112

Skin

   irritation 28-29

   problems 17

   ulcer 31

Sleep 18-19

Sleeping pills 51

Social support 99-100

Sodium valproate 40

Stress 41

Stroke 51

Sucking reflex 7

Sundowning 20,63

Sunlight 20

# INDEX

*Please use these following blank pages for your own notes and reminders.*

*All best wishes,*
*The Authors*